PHOBIAS

AND HOW TO

OVERCOME THEM

**Understanding and
Beating Your Fears**

PHOBIAS

AND HOW TO

OVERCOME THEM

Understanding and
Beating Your Fears

James Gardner, M.D., and Arthur H. Bell, Ph.D.

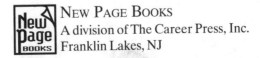

NEW PAGE BOOKS
A division of The Career Press, Inc.
Franklin Lakes, NJ

PHOBIAS AND HOW TO OVERCOME THEM
EDITED BY GINA M. CHESELKA
TYPESET BY KRISTEN PARKES
Cover design by Cheryl Cohan Finbow
Printed in the U.S.A. by Book-mart Press

To order this title, please call toll-free 1-800-CAREER-1 (NJ and Canada: 201-848-0310) to order using VISA or MasterCard, or for further information on books from Career Press.

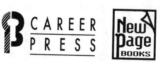

The Career Press, Inc., 3 Tice Road, PO Box 687,
Franklin Lakes, NJ 07417
www.careerpress.com
www.newpagebooks.com

Library of Congress Cataloging-in-Publication Data
Gardner, James, 1959-
    Phobias and how to overcome them : understanding and beating your fears / by James Gardner and Arthur H. Bell.
        p. cm.
    Includes bibliographical references and index.
    ISBN 1-56414-766-5 (paper)
    1. Phobias--Popular works. 2. Phobias--Treatment. I. Bell, Arthur H. (Arthur Henry), 1946- II. Title.

RC535.G37 2005
616.85'225--dc22

                                                                2004058359

DISCLAIMER

This book contains information that the authors believe to be correct. However, no recommendation for any individual's treatment, therapy, or medical care is intended, expressed, or implied. No reader should act on the basis of any printed medical information, including the contents of this book, without consultation with a health professional.

Dedication

FOR JAMES GARDNER, M.D.

This book is dedicated to my 18-month-old son, Jacob. Now that all the writing is complete, he can pluck the keys off my laptop and press the "delete" and "backspace" buttons all he wants. I can't wait to see his face when he realizes I am not an integral part of the ergonomic chair at my desk. With love and appreciation, I thank my wife, Patty; my mother-in-law, Julien Lin; my brother-in-law, Dr. Jackie Chen; and our long-time friend Chen Shihtang for their cooperation with my schedule and 24/7 loving care of Jacob.

FOR ARTHUR H. BELL, PH.D.

I dedicate my work with love to my wife, Dayle, and to my children, Art, Lauren, and Madeleine. They are in every sense my inspiration.

ACKNOWLEDGMENTS

For James Gardner, M.D.

In the preparation of this book, I drew on the experience and knowledge of my friends, family, patients, and respected colleagues. In addition to case details woven together and fictionalized for privacy from many chart records, many patients filled out an office questionnaire designed to elicit insights into the genesis and propagation of their individual phobic experiences. Their stories, again with changes made for the protection of privacy, became an important part of the fabric of this text.

Several specialists in the field of psychology and psychiatry were central to my understanding and appreciation of the complexity of this subject. I would like to especially thank Brent Cox, M.D.; William Barton, Ph.D.; Stephen Drew, Ph.D.; Stephen M. Stahl, M.D., Ph.D.; Jaime Nissenbaum, Ph.D.; Jeffrey Humpfries, M.D.; Michael Freeman, M.D.; and Michael Vurel, Ph.D.

Colleagues and personal friends in a variety of medical and surgical specialties generously answered my many questions about their personal experiences with phobias or working with patients suffering from anxiety and phobic conditions. They include Alan Pont, M.D.; Terry DuBrow, M.D.; Tanya Atagi, M.D.; Robert Aycock, M.D.; Robert Hines, M.D.; Richard Printz, M.D.; Linda Gaudiani, M.D.; Michael Moskowitz, M.D.; Ilkan Cokgor, M.D.; Julie Griffith, M.D.; Robert Belknap, M.D.; Peggy Skilling, RN; and Nina Titova, RPT. As always, my friend and attorney, John Truxaw, was helpful and supportive throughout this project.

My father, the Rev. T.F. Gardner, is appreciated for fielding theological questions regarding the effects of emotional disorders on health, healing, spirituality, and personal fulfillment.

As with our last project, *Overcoming Anxiety, Panic, and Depression* (New Page Books, 2000), Dr. Bell and I enjoyed a stimulating and enthusiastic collaboration that made the process seem effortless.

I hope the real experiences that were drawn upon to create this book will help our readers connect with their own phobic suffering and begin to move toward a more fearless and fulfilled future.

FOR ARTHUR H. BELL, PH.D.

As a speech coach and professor of management communication, I work with students, managers, and executives whose fears frequently get in the way of their intended performance. For his insights and expertise in addressing such fears, I owe deep gratitude to my coauthor, James Gardner, M.D. In addition, I send a general note of thanks to my professors at Harvard and the University of Southern California, as well as to my valued colleagues at USC, Georgetown University, and the University of San Francisco. A special thanks also goes to the more than 500 managers, lawyers, executives, and other professionals for whom I have had the privilege of serving as a presentation coach and mentor. Their varied experiences with the fear of public speaking gave me a lifelong scholarly interest in phobias, although not as a medical practitioner. I am also grateful to my wonderful friends and relatives for their many kindnesses and expressions of encouragement during the development of this book.

Both authors would like to thank the talented editors at New Page Books for their admirable work: Michael Pye, Gina Cheselka, Kristen Parkes, Kate Henches, and Stacey A. Farkas.

CONTENTS

PREFACE

Like our previous book together, *Overcoming Anxiety, Panic, and Depression* (New Page Books, 2000), this work focuses on you. We want the information, encouragement, alternatives, and insights in these pages to help free you from the burden of phobias and related fears.

Dozens of stories appear in this book (all thoroughly disguised and conflated, if from case files) to let you know that many, many other people have experienced what you are going through with phobias. These stories also reveal ways out of such suffering—and those ways differ significantly from person to person. Because our individual routes to recovery depend so much on our personalities, experiences, and even our genes, we have provided an entire "Anxiety Toolbox" in Chapter 9 to help you phase out your phobias as quickly as possible. Not uncommonly, a combination of tools succeeds where no one tool alone proves adequate.

In addition, Dr. Gardner, along with a staff of medical specialists and experts in a wide range of relevant fields, has taken the concept of the "Toolbox" further to create a comprehensive program to help those suffering from all forms of anxiety. It is called the "Anxiety Toolbox Program," and can be purchased as a download from *www.anxietytoolbox.com*. This Website offers descriptions of a wide range of anxiety symptoms and conditions, and explains how they can be conquered through an integrated strategy using tools from the Anxiety Toolbox. The download includes the Comprehensive Anxiety Screening Tool (CAST) self-test and the Personal Anxiety Assessment List (PAAL), both designed specifically for the Anxiety

Toolbox Program to help you identify anxiety conditions and organize a personalized anxiety-busting plan of attack.

This downloadable program will be useful not only to individuals with diagnosed anxiety disorders, but also to those who desire more control and success in their relationships and careers, those battling addictions and patterns of self-destructive behavior, and those who want to improve their performance in sports requiring mental focus and concentration. Gaining control over anxiety has been shown to improve overall physical health and brain function, enhancing memory, learning, and immune system responses. Also, recent studies have verified that the process of aging is accelerated by anxiety, creating a higher incidence of stroke and heart disease.

The Anxiety Toolbox Program provides the basic tools needed to defeat anxiety in a way that can be tailored to each person's diagnosis and individual sensibilities, and can easily be applied to even the most hectic lifestyle. The program is divided into eight compartments that teach "tried and true" strategies that are both primitive and high-tech, ancient and modern, Eastern and Western, modern medical and alternative, and psychotherapeutic and spiritual. Only those tools showing real benefit are presented. We hope this book and the unique online program will allow those with anxiety to find the inner peace and security that is the hallmark of emotional health.

We want to emphasize that this book and the Anxiety Toolbox Program are in no way substitutes for the advice and care of a skilled medical or psychological professional. Although general principles and practices of treatment are described here, no specific recommendation for any individual's therapy or medical care is intended, expressed, or implied. When it comes to health care, no reader should act on the basis of any printed information, including the contents of this book, without consultation with a health professional.

Above all, this book is a conversation between you and the authors—a conversation we hope will extend to your doctor, psychologist, or psychiatrist. Perhaps the topics, terms, and ideas you find in this book can help you formulate just what you want to say about your situation to your health professional.

To begin the conversation, let us introduce ourselves in our own voices.

"Hello, I'm Dr. James Gardner. For almost two decades I have practiced general medicine in Marin County, California. Of my present patient group of approximately 3,500, some 30 to 40 percent suffer from phobias, anxiety, panic, and depressive disorders, or some combination thereof. I see patients of all ages, ethnic backgrounds, educational levels, and social status. It has been my deep privilege to be intimately involved in their life experiences and care. I also serve as a clinical instructor at the School of Medicine, University of California at San Francisco and am a university lecturer on anxiety, depression, phobias, and the grief response."

"And hello from Art Bell. Although I am not a medical or psychological practitioner, I do lecture on speech and performance phobias and related anxieties in the M.B.A. and Executive M.B.A. programs at the University of San Francisco, where I am a professor of management communication and director of communication programs for the Masagung Graduate School of Business. For the past 20 years I have worked as a speech coach and management consultant for hundreds of business and government leaders. I hold my Ph.D. from Harvard University and am the author of 40 or so books in my field."

Conversations, of course, should be two-way in nature. We want to hear from you. Although we can't offer individual advice or counseling by e-mail, we do want to know what you have found helpful in this book or our previous publication. Contact Dr. Gardner at docgardner@anxietytoolbox.com and Art Bell at bell.a@sbcglobal.net.

James Gardner, M.D.
Greenbrae, California
August, 2004

Arthur H. Bell
Belvedere, California
August, 2004

Chapter 1

FACING YOUR PHOBIAS

This chapter answers five questions:

1. What is a phobia?
2. What are the most common phobias?
3. What does a severe phobic response feel like?
4. How do phobia sufferers typically seek relief?
5. Why do phobia sufferers often fail to see the whole picture?

Do you or does someone you care about suffer from phobias? If so, this book is for you. Here we explain what phobias are, where they come from, and—perhaps most important—what you can do about them.

We take phobias seriously as threats not so much to life itself (although sometimes they are), but as obstacles to *lifestyle*. Phobias prevent people from enjoying many activities, ranging from business or personal travel, to a nature walk, to simply swallowing bites of a delicious meal. And others who care about a phobic person suffer as well. When a husband can't cross bridges or drive on freeways, a wife must often stay at home as well or go alone. When a friend can't fly, reunions are postponed for months, then years. When a father fears water, a child misses splashing with Dad.

If the solution to phobias was easy and apparent, the problem wouldn't exist. Those burdened by phobias know that "willing them away" rarely works. And, in truth, no one sells a pill or markets a single technique guaranteed to remove phobic suffering for all people in all cases.

In this book we propose several answers to the dilemma of phobic suffering. One of these or several in combination may well set you on the right path for recovery. We emphasize up front that no one technique is an instant "miracle" cure. Getting over a phobia that has plagued a person for many years requires time, patience, and effort. In most cases, the assistance of a health professional is highly recommended to help you apply the recovery concepts and strategies of this book to your individual situation. As with many of life's most complicated issues, simply knowing about phobias does not in itself guarantee psychological healing. Your physician, psychologist, psychiatrist, or other mental health counselor can help you turn good ideas into life realities. We hope that those good ideas begin with your reading of these chapters.

You're in Good Company!

It may be some consolation that you are not alone in your experience of a phobia. In fact, many highly regarded and successful individuals throughout history have been afflicted by a wide variety of phobic conditions. Below is a short list of some notable personalities and their phobias, as recently listed in *U.S. News and World Report* (November 24, 2004):

- Napoleon Bonaparte: ailurophobia (fear of cats)
- Queen Elizabeth I: subtype of anthophobia (fear of roses)
- Sigmund Freud: agoraphobia (fear of having an anxiety attack in a situation where escape might be difficult or embarrassing, such as a public gathering place)
- Howard Hughes: mysophobia (fear of germs...nonetheless, he spent his final years so paralyzed by fear that he was isolated and lived in squalor)
- Edgar Allen Poe and Harry Houdini: claustrophobia (fear of small, crowded, or confined spaces)
- Andre Agassi: arachnophobia (fear of spiders)
- Donald Trump: chirophobia (fear of shaking hands)
- Cher, Whoopi Goldberg, John Madden, and Aretha Franklin: aviophobia (fear of flying)
- Paul Newman: social phobia (fear of social situations)
- Billy Bob Thornton: fear of antiques

WHAT IS A PHOBIA?

Phobia, stemming from the Greek word for "fear," names a special set of apprehensions, anxieties, and terrors tied to particular things, places, experiences, and situations. As we will see throughout the following chapters, the list of different kinds of phobias is as various as life itself. Documented cases of phobias have involved the fear of swallowing, fear of babies, fear of tall trees, fear of short people, fear of dark clouds, and fear of peanut butter sticking to the roof of one's mouth. The most common phobias by far are those related to flying; snakes; insects; heights; enclosure; crowds; hypodermic needles; and functions and status of the body, including illnesses, blood, and injury.

You probably do not need to consult a book to know if you suffer from a particular phobia. The phobic experience is memorable indeed, standing out as a giant emotional spike in the usual ups and downs of daily life. For example, Calvin begins his day with his usual set of feelings, issues, and hang-ups. He groans when he steps on the scale and worries that his new diet isn't working. He makes small talk with his girlfriend at breakfast and worries that the relationship is fading. He starts his car and worries that the ping in the engine means a big repair bill in the near future. These are the common stressors and anxieties of daily living.

But when Calvin enters the East Tunnel, an emotional spike occurs that differs in intensity, symptoms, and painfulness from his normal emotional life. When the traffic stops dead at the bottom of the tunnel, Calvin feels suddenly overwhelmed by his long-standing phobia of tunnels, particularly the feeling of being trapped in a tunnel. He begins to sweat profusely, his pulse rate soars, and panic sets in. He grips his steering wheel with white knuckles. Only when traffic begins to move again and Calvin is free of the tunnel and back into the daylight does his composure begin, slowly, to return. Exhausted, he feels he has been to hell and back—and vows to avoid tunnels at all costs in the future.

Calvin's experience qualifies as a classic case of phobia because his intense fears are aroused by the presence of a particular thing or experience—the tunnel in this case—and are alleviated only when that stimulus is removed. In this sense, phobias can be viewed as the hot peppers in the salad of life. You have no doubts when you experience them, nor do you confuse them with run-of-the-mill anxieties of life.

THE FUNNY SIDE OF PHOBIAS

In an era and culture sensitive to most forms of mental and emotional illness, it's ironic that we continue to find phobias—the phobias of others, of course—somewhat humorous and entertaining. Usually we do not joke about the physical or emotional infirmities of others; Lord Byron's crippled foot, Winston Churchill's lisp, or John F. Kennedy's back problems aren't subjects available for jest. Yet when it comes to phobias, we as a culture seem to take relish in entertaining stories about the seemingly quaint fears of others. There is a part of us, as a culture, that likes to hear about Fred's morbid fear of spiders, Mabel's dread of deep water, and John's anxiety over germs on his hands. Such anecdotes are sufficiently exotic—that is, unlike our own experiences—to fascinate us.

At the same time, these stories increase our own sense of elevated status in relation to Fred, Mabel, and John. We feel "one up" because we do not suffer from these specific phobias. We enhance our own status by branding and labeling Fred, Mabel, and John in our own minds with their particular fears so that when we think of these people it is never without some thought to their phobic problems. Like the classic cartoon of the rich man slipping head over heels on a banana peel, we deflate others—albeit humorously—by picturing them forever being tripped up by the banana peel of their phobias.

We find some phobias so unusual and outright ridiculous, in fact, that we can't imagine why Fred, Mabel, and John don't break out laughing at their own fears. Take Fred, for example. He's a mesomorphic specimen with muscles on top of muscles, yet he can be reduced to a puddle of trembling perspiration by a small, nonpoisonous spider crawling across his desk.

Absurd? Not to Fred. And that's the key message with regard to any humor or entertainment we may find in the seemingly bizarre fears of others: their fears are as real to them as a crippled foot, lisp, or back problem. A culture of ridicule forces phobia sufferers to hide their dilemmas and, at the moment of a phobic episode, to worry about negative judgments and pointed fingers from others. In truth, there's nothing funny about phobias to those who suffer from them.

HOW PHOBIA SUFFERERS SEEK RELIEF

You may wonder what in the world Calvin was doing in the East Tunnel when he knew full well that he suffered from a tunnel phobia. In fact,

Calvin is not atypical of the large percentage of phobia sufferers who attempt to get over their fears by putting themselves again and again in the feared situation. They may rationalize that they have to cross a bridge or drive through a tunnel to get to work. But the underlying "script" being enacted here goes something like this: "I'm being silly to freak out in this tunnel. Thousands of people pass safely through it every day. I'm not going to let my ridiculous fears get the best of me. I can drive through this tunnel as confidently as anyone else. I just have to force myself to do it."

The notion of forcing oneself to overcome phobias helps to explain why so many phobic sufferers end up so often in exactly the circumstances they fear most—facing the barking dog, sitting on a crowded bus, swimming in deep water, and so forth. They push themselves to repeatedly experience their phobia in the hope (sometimes the misguided hope) that repeated suffering will eventually bring relief. Although some people do overcome phobias in this way, many others discover that touching a hot stove hurts just as much the 100th time as it did the first—and all the more so, if increasing injury (in the case of phobias, psychological injury) makes the pain worse.

Other phobic sufferers beat a quick path to their physician for a checkup. Too often in these few minutes of medical counsel the patient fails to tell the whole story of the phobic episode, sometimes out of embarrassment and sometimes from a lack of comprehension of the disorienting, frightening phobic event. For example, a patient fresh from a phobic episode may tell his physician that "sometimes my heart races and I feel clammy" instead of recounting the whole circumstance of the tunnel, the stopped traffic, and the onset of panic. With the best of professional intentions, a physician may give the patient a thorough physical exam and pronounce, with the goal of reassurance, that "you're perfectly fine."

Thousands of phobic sufferers come out of such doctor appointments only to be more confused than ever by their next phobic experience: "My heart is supposedly okay, but why is it racing again when I enter the tunnel? Why do I feel light-headed?" Many of these people seek further medical testing, second opinions, and advanced diagnosis in the hope of discovering "what's wrong with me."

Those who do tell their phobia story clearly to their physician may also encounter obstacles. Their doctor may recognize that a phobia is the likely cause of the patient's symptoms, but the physician may not be prepared to undertake time-consuming, talk-oriented therapy to address the problem.

In an era of HMOs, PPOs, and "capitation" (in which a participating physician is financially pressured to limit outside referrals), the doctor may not make it a practice to send phobia sufferers promptly to a mental health professional for help. The doctor may remark, "You may want to see a psychologist or psychiatrist," with the subtext inferred by the patient, *"...if you really think you are crazy."* The doctor sometimes fails to suggest names and make a specific referral. Many phobia sufferers, already confused and discouraged by their situation, do not have the moxie or information resources to seek out a mental health professional on their own.

Another group of phobia sufferers attempt to self-medicate their way to relief, most commonly with alcohol ("a stiff drink usually gets me through"), nicotine ("I'm okay if I can smoke"), and tranquilizers such as Ativan ("atta-boy"), Xanax, Valium, and their kin. For example, the senior manager who fears public speaking gets his courage up with a couple shots of whiskey before the big speech and drowns his sorrows after the speech with more alcohol. The interior designer who fears bridges pacifies herself by taking Ativan, which she purchases 30 pills at a time for $169 from an Internet pharmacy in Canada after her physician refused to renew her prescription. The obvious risks of substance addiction and abuse in these cases significantly outweigh any physical danger from phobic reactions.

Finally, the largest percentage of phobia sufferers self-treat their illness by avoidance of the feared thing or experience. Calvin quits his job to find work where he will never have to enter a tunnel. Those who fear dogs sell their homes to find apartments in dog-prohibited buildings. Those who fear snakes or particular insects move hundreds or thousands of miles away in search of a phobia-free existence. In the process, these people discover, first, that phobic stimuli are hard to avoid entirely; and second, that the extinguishment of one phobia through avoidance may simply be the prelude to a new phobia. For example, the woman who moves to San Francisco to avoid thunderstorms (San Francisco has very few) may find that she begins to fear some other weather phenomenon, such as blinding fog (of which San Francisco has an abundance). A person's psychological need for a phobia of some kind is rarely dissolved by avoidance alone.

PHOBIAS AND SOCIAL EMBARRASSMENT

A significant portion of the suffering accompanying phobic fears stems not from actual terror over the mold spores on the orange, slithering coils of the snake, or possibility of choking on a bite of steak, but on what others will think. Depending on our desire for approval and general social needs, we may go to great lengths to hide our phobic responses or to avoid situations that we feel may bring on such reactions. For example, a commercial real estate broker who fears heights may struggle mightily with impending feelings of panic as he shows an upper-story office suite with a suspended balcony overlooking the city. He may avoid such situations entirely, to his financial disadvantage and the befuddlement of his boss and clients.

The fear of what others will think—in itself a possible form of phobia—can intensify the sensations associated with a phobic episode. Worrying about the reactions of others becomes a pressure cooker for the person experiencing a phobic episode. It's one thing for Linda, a grade-school teacher, to stay out of the reptile house when she takes her class on a field trip to the zoo, with the explanation "I just hate snakes." But it's quite another thing when she attempts to hide her fear of snakes, under the assumption that her students and their parents will think less of her if she appears unable to lead a cage-by-cage, scale-by-scale tour of the reptile house.

Picture Linda's agony due to her fear not only of snakes, but of social embarrassment as well. She begins to perspire as she nears the cool, dark entrance to the reptile house. She feels strangely unsteady and light-headed as the first snake specimen comes into view. Sensations of panic wash across her as she tries to keep up her docent talk on the wonders of snakes, while all the time feeling an overpowering need to rush out of the reptile house. She worries that her physical discomfort and growing sense of terror must be apparent to those around her. She interprets the glance of any student or parent as the question, "Teacher, are you okay?" She bears down with all her might to fight against her emotions of fear, intensified now by her anxiety over what others are thinking about her. At last, drenched in sweat and weak from her emotional wars, she stumbles out the exit door of the reptile house, vowing silently *never again!* when it comes to leading field trips to the zoo.

How can the pressure cooker of others' reactions be turned off? Being honest with others about what you can and can't do certainly has general merit. Social anxiety can be relieved when others know about and accept your limitations. Self-acceptance of such limitations can also be a step toward internal peace.

But an important caveat or footnote should accompany any blanket advice to simply accept and admit one's perceived limitations. It's deceptively easy to assert that phobic sufferers should simply announce their handicaps to others and let the chips fall where they may. In many situations, phobic sufferers don't want to give in to their phobias. They see others having fun at a particular activity and they want to enjoy the activity as well. In addition, they know that the convenience and pleasure of others is directly impacted by the phobic person's problems. A husband, Bob, hates to let his wife down by passing up an opportunity for an anniversary cruise to Alaska all because he has experienced a long-standing fear of being at sea. In this case, Bob's love for his wife conflicts directly with his accommodation to his phobia. Part of him may want to nix the whole idea of a cruise, but another part of him would like to see his wife enjoy the time of her life on a long-anticipated cruise.

Bob also knows from personal experience that phobias often rise and fall in intensity, with the sufferer experiencing "good days and bad days." For this reason, many phobic sufferers find themselves taking a chance on life experiences that may trigger their fears. They end up in phobic struggles not because they were too unaware to predict and avoid these situations, but because they a) weren't positive that their phobias would occur, in which case they could enjoy the activity at hand; and b) they didn't want to disappoint others who counted on their companionship and/or participation.

So we find Bob on the third day at sea, stuck in the middle of an agonizing phobic episode. He lies on an examining table in the ship's infirmary, a basket case of nerves and insomnia. He is upset not only by his familiar phobic symptoms having to do with sea travel, but all the more mortified by his failure to help his wife enjoy their "dream vacation." She may sit by his side and pat his hand reassuringly, but in his heart of hearts he deeply regrets disappointing her (though she tells him she is not disappointed). What will they tell others about their trip when they return? Bob is experiencing fear not just over the possibility but also over the actuality of ruining his wife's trip. He has been emotionally burned by risking sea travel, with the result that his sea phobia takes a deeper and more permanent hold over his living. His anguish reminds him that "I can't fight this thing. I was stupid to try. I have to avoid being at sea at all costs."

The social costs of phobic suffering are real and complex. They cannot be wished away by a "just be honest to others" policy. Oversimplifying the impact of one's phobia on others ("Don't worry, others will understand") can backfire when the phobic sufferer faces situations where significant others are disappointed, are confused, and are themselves frightened by the sudden onset of a friend's or loved one's phobic episode. Pretending otherwise gives a "get out of jail free" card to the phobic sufferer, enabling him or her to nourish and surrender to the very phobia that threatens his or her fulfillment. However painful to experience, the social embarrassment occasioned by phobic suffering may sometimes turn out to be a healthful and powerful antidote to self-absorption in one's phobic dilemma. The disappointment, concern, and fright of others is their way of expressing their wish that things could be otherwise. That same wish should become the agenda of anyone seeking freedom from their phobias.

PHOBIAS AND THE IMAGINED WORST-CASE SCENARIO

Jefferson, a middle-aged banker, tells his psychologist about his worsening fear of lightning:

"It sounds ridiculous, I know, but I am starting to avoid business trips to any location where thunderstorms typically occur. I'm especially terrified at the prospect of seeing lightning during an airline flight or passing near thunderheads where lightning might strike the plane. If I'm at home or at a hotel during a rainstorm, I won't even go out to catch a cab. I can't tell you how many business meetings I've missed at the last minute because of my fear of lightning. I make up flimsy excuses, usually having to do with migraine headaches or the sudden illness of a relative. But, bottom line, this phobia is messing up my life."

Jefferson knows, of course, that his chances of being struck by lightning are infinitely less than his chances, let's say, of dying in an automobile crash.

"Statistics don't help," Jefferson counters. "I would be just as afraid if my chances were one in a billion instead of one in a million or one in a thousand."

At the core of Jefferson's phobia—and, by extension, many other phobias—is the sufferer's perception of the imagined worst-case scenario. Getting the phobic sufferer to express this scenario in detail can give a mental health counselor and the sufferer himself significant insight into the nature and eventual extinguishment of the phobia at hand.

What exactly does Jefferson fear? In his mind, what is the worst that will happen if he does not obsessively avoid all circumstances even marginally related to lightning? Jefferson explains:

"I picture something like this as my worst-case scenario: I know that dark clouds are gathering, but I take a chance and step outside just to get a newspaper or catch a cab. I walk quickly for a few steps and nothing happens. But just before I reach safety in the form of a cab or in returning to my home or hotel, I'm struck by an incredibly powerful electric jolt that sends my eyes popping from their sockets and sizzles my internal organs. I picture myself a convict in the electric chair, with smoke rising from my ears and mouth. I don't die immediately, but lie there without anyone to help me, feeling my heart in its last convulsions. In my death throes, I'm thinking how I knew this would happen and how I should never have taken the risk. I should have played it safe. The lightning was just waiting to get me and I gave it the opportunity. Now I paid the price and would never have a second chance. My life was over because I just wasn't careful enough."

Without overanalyzing Jefferson's phobia, it is apparent that he fears more than the physical phenomenon of lightning. He associates lightning with any severe, painful punishment or attack that comes "out of the blue" without warning and without remorse. Here is the fearful child hiding in fear of an inexplicable blow from an angry parent. Here is the cave dweller at risk of sudden assault from a beast of prey.

The worst-case scenario for Jefferson is doing the wrong thing, making the wrong move, and thereby leaving himself defenseless to the dragon just outside the door. He believes that sudden, horribly painful tragedy lurks for him as his fate in life. The only option he perceives lies in retreat, hiding, and excuses. He feels ashamed by taking this route, and therefore views himself as all the more fated for a sudden strike of punishment. His worst-case scenario is for "it" to happen, symbolically in the form of lightning, but more realistically in the form of some devastating life event, such as terminal illness, unexpected divorce, financial disaster, or the death of a loved one. Jefferson fears most what he cannot control. At the same time, he realizes that living in minute-by-minute expectation of disaster is no life at all.

Phobias teased out to the sticking point of their worst-case scenario often provide this kind of reflective material for personal growth and decision-making. The subjects of our phobias, whether lightning or lightning bugs, can tell us much about our deeper, more essential concerns when they are viewed as symbolic stand-ins—lightning rods, as it were. As suggested later in this book, a phobic sufferer can learn much about the deeper nature of his or her fears by keeping a journal or writing down descriptions of not only the fears themselves, but also the surrounding thoughts and impressions that accompany those fears.

HEARING THE PART OF THE STORY YOU
WOULD LIKE TO SKIP

Many phobic sufferers believe they have their whole situation figured out in advance of seeing a health care professional or, for that matter, reading a book on phobias. They have their own theory of where their phobias came from, their own plan for dealing with them, and their own prognosis for eventual recovery. Breaking into that airtight world with valuable new information can be difficult.

For example, a phobic sufferer who is sure that his phobia is a failure of character or a sign of emotional instability may have little interest in the chapters of this book dealing with the physical basis of many phobias. The person who experiences phobias as the "black sheep" from supposedly perfect parents may not want to learn in Chapter 2 about the hereditary nature of many common phobias. A person who pooh-poohs his phobia may not want to read in Chapter 6 about the frequent links between phobic suffering and underlying depressive disorders. And certainly, the person who moans and groans about his phobia to all who will listen may not want to read in Chapter 3 about the subtle love affair we often have with phobias that bedevil us.

Any phobic sufferer must assume at the outset that he or she is not seeing an important part of the picture. Like any neurosis, a phobia by definition involves a distorted perception of what others see as common reality. A person who sees every dog as a death threat has to be open to information that challenges and ultimately revises that view of the world. Therefore, we urge those plagued by phobias to take special interest in precisely those portions of this book that they don't believe to be immediately applicable. In effect, a reader can say, "I know I have a tendency to see things through the filter of my phobia. To escape that distorted vision, I need to be open-minded about new ideas, perspectives, and recovery techniques. If my old vision of things were enough, I would have already recovered from my phobia."

SUMMING UP AND LOOKING FORWARD

Phobias are irrational, dysfunctional, and unhelpful fear responses. The different phobias that have been identified and classified span the range of human experience and imagination. Because of the unpleasant physical symptoms that accompany these responses, avoidance of the feared subject, activity, or situation is a natural consequence. Whether standing alone as a specific phobia, triggered by the social interaction of social phobia as seen in the maladaptive fear and avoidance of agoraphobia (the fear and avoidance of places or situations where the individual believes they may experience anxiety symptoms that could result in embarrassment, incapacitation, or some other catastrophe), or arising from an underlying anxiety disorder, phobias can be anything from mildly annoying to deeply painful and embarrassing experiences. In some cases, they can have a devastating effect on a person's career, relationships, and quality of life. Depression, alcoholism, drug use, divorce, and suicide are some of the more dramatic results of untreated phobias and their underlying anxiety conditions.

But much more common and often unrecognized are other, more subtle manifestations: a marriage that isn't fun anymore because of a partner's fears and anxieties; a career that stagnates and declines because of obstacles related to phobias; a timid and insecure personality focused on phobias instead of on opportunities for joy and passion. If untreated, phobias may limit our lives, often causing low self-esteem and poor self-confidence. In addition, because we do not live in a vacuum, our phobic dysfunctions can affect everyone around us: family, friends, and coworkers. This devastating influence on others is the "rest of the story" rarely told by phobia sufferers, focused as they are on their own fears. They are talkative about how they have suffered, but too often silent about the suffering they have brought to others.

Taking responsibility for phobias that block our way in life is an act of kindness that improves the lives of those who care about us. Freedom from phobias allows us to turn the focus outward and experience the fun of life. This book will teach various ways to understand and work with your nervous system to stop your phobic fear response and see the world afresh. It is a journey to a place of inner peace—in effect, a phobia-free zone.

Chapter 2

WHERE DO PHOBIAS COME FROM?

This chapter answers six questions:

1. Where do phobias come from?
2. Why doesn't my emotional mind obey my rational mind?
3. What underlying anxiety disorders can contribute to phobias?
4. What are the various ways in which phobias are experienced?
5. How do some people, often unknowingly, cling to their phobias for social and personal benefits?
6. Why should I have a healthy respect for the human fear mechanism?

Many people remember clearly the moment their phobia started. A painful, frightening, or embarrassing experience in youth is often to blame. For example, Mary remembers vividly how, at age 8, her neighborhood friends thought it would be fun to roll her up in a carpet and send her spinning down the driveway. Since then, she has a phobia related to small, closed-in spaces and has experienced many anxiety attacks in such situations.

For another patient, Judy, the phobia started in adulthood while traveling on a small commercial airplane. The low flight was especially bumpy, and panic set in when she looked down and saw a man barbecuing in his yard below. She was sure the plane was flying too low and would soon crash.

During the rest of the flight, Judy lay curled up in a tight ball on the floor. Her elevated heart rate and nausea persisted for a long time after deplaning.

RATIONAL AND EMOTIONAL REALITIES

These examples illustrate a fundamental point that will be the basis of our behavioral treatment strategies later in this book and in the companion Anxiety Toolbox Program (available online at *www.anxietytoolbox.com*). As humans, we process and learn information in two ways: rationally and emotionally. Our emotional reaction depends to some degree on the personality with which we're born. Timid and melancholy personalities have been found to be more vulnerable to anxiety and phobias than cheerful or bold personalities. In addition, early life experiences and beliefs cause us to make generalizations that we then apply to later situations.

This application of the past to the present and future is the automatic, adaptive, and "smart" way of processing information described by Seymour Epstein and Archie Brodsky in their book *You're Smarter Than You Think* (Simon & Schuster, 1993). Unfortunately, our emotional mode of processing past feelings and information sometimes contains unhelpful elements, such as irrational fears. These fears are not based on reality, but on how we *interpret* events and information. For example, almost all of us remember a time when we were fearful of monsters living under the bed or in the closet. As we got older, these misinterpretations of our world were corrected by our rational minds. Our emotions were guided by our rationality.

But until rational thoughts exercise a calming and ordering effect on the emotions, we, like Mary and Judy, can continue to relive frightening emotional moments. Rolled up in the carpet, Mary felt trapped and unable to control her situation. Her adaptive, emotional mode of learning informed her that, in the future, she had to beware of any closed-in space. Such a situation, her emotions told her, would cause her to feel vulnerable and possibly to lose control. The same anxiety she experienced while bound up inside the restrictive roll of carpet would immediately reoccur if she gets in an elevator or any small space where escape might be difficult. Even sitting toward the middle of a long row of theater seats, where she could not easily leave, caused Mary's feelings of panic to rise.

Because of Mary's specific phobia to closed-in spaces (claustrophobia), she avoids a number of potential situations or activities that might involve being confined or restricted. She won't enjoy a ride in the amusement park or take a crowded bus because she fears having an anxiety attack that will be simultaneously frightening and humiliating. This avoidance behavior resulting from her fear of having a symptom attack is the hallmark of agoraphobia, discussed in detail in Chapter 5.

Like Mary, Judy also had an upsetting emotional experience (hers on the low-flying plane), but it was caused in large part by her rational mind being misinformed. Not being an experienced traveler, she overestimated the level of danger presented by turbulence and low altitude. She did not know that smaller planes often fly much lower than the larger jets she was familiar with. A "Fear of Flying Clinic" helped her understand the mechanics of flight and appreciate the safety record of commercial airlines, which was an important aspect of her successful recovery.

LEARNING AND UNLEARNING OUR FEAR RESPONSES

Both rational and emotional modes of learning can sometimes conspire to amplify our fear responses. Dave was a patient who developed a phobia concerning his health (hypochondriasis) after he thought he was dying from a heart attack. He had learned from a half-baked TV program that chest pain always means a life-threatening catastrophe is at hand. So when he experienced what turned out to be simple heartburn, he was quite concerned. The more he worried, the worse the discomfort became. He pressed his wrist and neck and noticed that his heart rate was elevated. He felt sweaty and faint.

He turned, now feeling desperate, to the Web for medical information only to find lists of cardiac symptoms that increased his alarm. Now truly terrified, he called 911 and was taken to the ER for what turned out to be an acute anxiety attack. After a normal EKG and lab tests, Dave was sent home with no explanation of what had happened. "You're fine," the doctor said as he rushed to the next patient. Nurses gave Dave a patronizing smile and pat on the shoulder, but no information.

In this case, the ER doctor was too busy to give Dave's rational mind a full explanation and discussion of the physiology of anxiety attacks. Without this reassurance, Dave went home wondering if his "heart symptoms" simply didn't show up in the hospital or if the ER doctor had examined him too casually (the Internet had given Dave enough information about ER doctors to doubt their expertise in more subtle aspects of cardiac care).

With all these questions active in his mind, Dave began fearing that any signal from his body—a twinge in his shoulder, a bout of indigestion, an occasional feeling of fatigue—was something to fret about to the point of experiencing panic attacks. Only after a process of cognitive unlearning about the reality of his bodily feelings was Dave's rational mind able to ignore his minor internal sensations without triggering an anxiety attack.

PHOBIAS AND UNDERLYING ANXIETY DISORDERS

As we will see in more detail in Chapter 6, many phobias arise in individuals who process information inaccurately due to an underlying anxiety disorder. These disorders are often inherited or come about because of an extreme stress or trauma. Panic disorder, post-traumatic stress disorder, generalized anxiety disorder, and obsessive-compulsive disorder are all diagnoses that must be treated to successfully make progress in extinguishing phobias and related fears.

For a person with an underlying anxiety disorder, any life stressor that causes his or her nervous system to be "on edge"—a divorce, a friend's unexpected death, legal problems, a letter from the IRS, job loss, or academic failure—can stimulate overreaction of the fear response and trigger a phobia or anxiety problem. Personality disorders, especially paranoid, avoidant, histrionic, narcissistic, and borderline personality types have been linked to a higher incidence of phobic disorders.

Not uncommonly, people with anxiety disorders have attempted, often for years, to "cope" with their emotions by chemical means. But drug use, including marijuana, amphetamines, and hallucinogens, invariably makes the nervous system more vulnerable to emotional disturbances such as phobias. Alcohol, perhaps the most common substance used for self-medication, usually makes phobias and anxiety worse by interfering with sleep patterns and creating further social and legal stressors.

Many other underlying or background emotional and physical factors can set the stage for a vulnerability to phobias. Children who were abused, neglected, or exposed to a particularly nervous and overreactive parent can often be expected to develop dysfunctional anxiety and phobic responses throughout life. Many medical conditions, including hormonal imbalances, chronic pain, depression, head trauma, thyroid disorders, sleep disorders, migraine headaches, diabetes, hypoglycemia, chronic fatigue, and autoimmune diseases such as lupus and fibromyalgia can weaken emotional health and open the door to phobia. In addition, many medications may act to increase anxious feelings. Among the most common of these medications are steroids, thyroid drugs, antidepressants, diet pills, and inhalers for asthma. Some over-the-counter supplements and stimulants, including decongestants, caffeinated products, and some herbal remedies can also be culprits in pushing a person toward phobic feelings. Finally, stress, emotional trauma, medical conditions, and genetic predispositions all play a role in causing an imbalance in our brain chemistry and increasing the number of overreactive receptors on our brain cells. All these factors create a fertile ground for the development of a phobic reaction.

In sum, phobias are now viewed as a natural and expected manifestation of an imbalance in the nervous system. They are compounded and aggravated by misinformation and misinterpretation of the experience by the individual. We call this imbalance in the nervous system "psychological sensitivity," which is influenced by:

1. Life experiences and trauma.

2. Personality type.

3. Underlying mood, anxiety, or behavioral disorders.

4. Unhealthy activities and lifestyle choices.

5. Underlying medical problems.

6. Lack of support and poor coping skills and strategies.

These factors will be discussed more completely in Chapter 7.

WHAT DOES A PHOBIA FEEL LIKE?

Even if two people share the same type of phobia—fear of frogs, let's say—Person A will no doubt experience that phobia somewhat differently than Person B (there is no such thing as *the* fear response to frogs). Yet if we were to catalog and compare what a phobia feels like "inside" to hundreds of people, we would discover not hundreds of completely distinct reactions to phobias, but instead some general areas of similarity.

These commonalities of response should not surprise us. We human beings share quite similar physiologies—normal temperature at 98.6° F, blood chemistry within the same narrow limits, and so forth. We also share somewhat similar psychologies, with Mom and Dad (and perhaps siblings and ex-spouses) figuring large in the background. No wonder that we are not absolutely individualistic in the ways we experience phobias. Admittedly, the fears associated with phobias can make an individual feel as if "no one understands what I am feeling." But when an individual discloses his or her phobic feelings and symptoms to others in, let's say, a group therapy session, that person commonly discovers that others have indeed had roughly similar feelings. It can be a relief, in fact, to realize that perhaps hundreds of thousands of people know through personal experience exactly what "your" phobic response feels like.

A VARIETY OF PHOBIC RESPONSES

Some people experience phobias primarily in terms of physical sensations: "I felt like I was suffocating...my heart was beating wildly...I was sweating profusely...I felt light-headed and dizzy...I became suddenly nauseous and clammy all over...my hands were shaking and all my muscles felt trembly...my cheeks felt blazing hot...my knees felt like they were going to buckle...." Often these physical sensations beget secondary cycles of fear, to the point that the original stimulus (frogs, remember?) can almost be lost sight of as a person focuses on dreaded physical discomforts.

Other people experience phobias as mental images, thoughts, or "voices": "My thoughts were racing out of my control...all I could picture was the fierce look in the dog's eyes...I felt like everyone in the room was staring at me...I could practically hear them asking what was wrong with me...the words 'you're going crazy, you're going crazy' kept recurring inside...I kept hearing my father saying 'Don't be silly, get hold of yourself,' but I just couldn't...all I could think was 'You're miles from any medical help; no one can come to your rescue.'"

Like physical feelings, these mental sensations can in themselves be frightening. As one patient said, "I knew I was just scaring myself by thinking negative and threatening thoughts, but I couldn't help myself. My thoughts seemed to have a life of their own. I was being attacked by my own thinking—and what could be more frightening and appalling than that?"

Still other people experience phobias in an emotional way, with the primary focus not on physical discomforts or specific thoughts, but instead on powerful if somewhat vague feelings: "I don't know how to describe it...I just felt absolute dread, as if I were going to die at any minute...I felt an overpowering need to get out of the auditorium right away...I just felt a wave of deep hopelessness...I felt spacy and weird, as if I was kind of detached from my body...I felt afraid, and my feelings kept building second by second...I thought I would explode."

Part of the frustration of experiencing phobias in an emotional way is the difficulty of communicating those feelings to others, including your physician, psychiatrist, or psychologist. Patients often preface their attempts at such communications by saying, "I don't know how to describe what I was feeling" or "It just came over me...I don't know what happened." Their inability to get a firm grasp on their phobic experiences can be an additional source of fear. The unknown and inexpressible aspects of these experiences can seem like an external, alien force that times simply takes command of consciousness and rationality at unpredictable times.

DETERMINING YOUR FEAR RESPONSE

Unfortunately, those who suffer phobic fears do not get to choose "door one, door two, or door three" to determine whether their fears will be experienced physically, mentally, or emotionally. Partly by nature and partly by nurture, we each are predisposed to interpret experience, including frightening experience, through a combination of sensations, often with one aspect (physical, mental, or emotional) being dominant. For example, a person may play through negative scripts mentally ("I will choke if I breathe dust, I will choke, I will choke") that lead to physical sensations (constricted airways, as in the case of stress-induced asthma) and emotional responses (anxiety and anguish). These sensations can occur simultaneously or, just as often, in a causal sequence (frightening thoughts perhaps occurring first, followed by emotional and physical sensations).

The feelings associated with phobias also run the gamut of intensity, from barely discernible and subtly irritating to severe and functionally paralyzing. In some cases a phobia "comes on strong" at its first occurrence (let's say a sudden attack of claustrophobia in a hot, crowded bus) and gradually subsides in intensity as the person learns to watch out for places and circumstances that bring on such feelings. Or a phobia can initially be felt as a slight, unexpected physical or emotional irritation—a bit of dizziness, for example, at the head of a flight of stairs—that grows stronger day by day as the person returns to the same location or situation.

In short, the answer to the question "What does a phobia feel like?" is highly individual, but not exclusively individual. In describing one's phobic feelings to a group of fellow sufferers, the chances are good that more than one person in the group will nod as if to say, "I've felt that same thing." Phobic sufferers should know in advance—and be reassured in knowing—that their description of symptoms, however halting or vague, will be familiar to their doctors and to those who have experienced anxiety attacks in one form or another.

PHOBIAS AND SOCIALLY ACCEPTABLE FEARS

Sometimes we like to scare ourselves, so long as the conditions for such fright events are thoroughly under our control. Take, for example, the obvious terror involved in being pursued by a Frankenstein-like monster obsessed with tearing us limb from limb. Virtually no one would choose such an experience in real life. We would not purposely put ourselves in harm's way without knowing how things will turn out. But millions of us will fork over the price of a movie ticket or click onto a TV movie to see all manner of demons, monsters, and madmen leap out of the screen at us (or at the movie stars with whom we identify).

People around the world choose to experience raw terror "at a distance"— in comfortable theater seats with their favorite snacks in hand—through movies ranging from *Night of the Living Dead* and *Friday the 13th* to *Jaws* and *Psycho*. If we understand the pleasure factor hidden within these cinematic terror experiences, we may have a better grasp of the staying power of some phobias in our lives and our inability to conquer them once and for all.

FRIGHT AS A SOCIAL ATTRACTOR

Picture Wendy contemplating whether to spend $9.00 to see *The Creature* on Saturday night. She shivers at the thought of going alone (such movies deeply frighten her and often result in recurring nightmares). She tells her sister, "Going alone to a horror flick just isn't any fun."

But when Walter calls to invite her to see the movie, the prospects change significantly, and not just because Walter will pay for the tickets. "It will be great," Wendy confides. "If I scream or grab Walter's arm, he will think it's really funny. And we will probably sit with a bunch of our friends. We'll get a pizza after the movie and talk about how weird the creature was and how it made us feel."

At the same time, Walter is telling his pals "It's cool to take a girl to a horror movie. They huddle up close to you during the scary parts and there's always something to talk about after the movie—like how scared they got and at what point in the movie they felt like they were going to freak out. Girls like to talk about that stuff."

The date goes well, and both Wendy and Walter conclude that horror movies are "their thing." Although they are rather shy and timid in real life, they nevertheless seek out terrifying movie experiences to enjoy together. In short, they choose fright in limited doses for what it does for them socially.

CHERISHING THE PHOBIAS WE CLAIM TO HATE

We can apply these insights to an understanding of some (but certainly not all) phobias. As odd as it may seem at first, some people cherish their pet phobias for the social dividends these fears pay. Consider the case of Anita's feather phobia:

"As a young child growing up on a farm, I had to gather eggs each day from our chickens. One time the door to the chicken coop got stuck and I found myself locked up for almost an hour with a bunch of increasingly agitated hens and roosters. All I really remember is all the feathers floating in the air and the horrible feeling that I couldn't breathe. Ever since, I get panicky when I'm too close to loose feathers, even from fluffing up a feather pillow."

Anita has told this story to every one of her friends and acquaintances at her bridge club. In turn, many of these people have shared their own stories of early childhood frights. In the process they have bonded more closely with one another. Friends sometimes use their knowledge of Anita's feather phobia to express caring and kindness for her ("Anita, I was thinking of wearing my hat with the feathers to the charity banquet, but I certainly won't if it will bother you"). Anita assures her friends that only loose feathers cause her discomfort and thank them for being considerate.

Similarly, Anita's husband "earns points" by catering to Anita's phobia. When they travel on vacation, Al makes a point of telling the hotel reservations clerk that "We need synthetic pillows. My wife is allergic to feathers." Of course, Anita is not literally allergic to feathers, but she appreciates her husband's euphemism that spares her the embarrassment of explaining her feather fears to a stranger. Serving Anita's phobic needs in ways large and small becomes one of the ways by which Al shows himself to be a loving husband (and in turn reaps the rewards, such as they are, that come due to loving husbands).

CHOOSING THE PHOBIA OF OUR HEART'S DESIRE

In analyzing Anita's feather phobia, we should distinguish between historical fact and convenient emotional fiction. It is a fact that as a young child Anita was frightened by her accidental lockup with flapping chickens, an experience that she has remembered as feathers floating all around her and a choking inability to breathe born of panic. But Anita, like most of us, had dozens of frightening experiences in childhood—being chased by a dog, falling from a tree limb, choking on food, jumping at a clap of thunder, and so forth. Out of all these frightening experiences, why has she settled on feathers as the preferred phobia to which she, her husband, and her friends give frequent attention? Why has the feather phobia become Anita's personal houseplant for daily watering and emotional fertilization?

We can answer this question by considering Anita's life without her pet phobia. At her bridge club, Anita—a somewhat bland person, truth be told—without her fear of feathers would have one less special thing to distinguish her from everyone else. She would have one less disclosing story to confide as a way of gaining the interest and friendship of others. In her marital life, Anita would give up one reliable point of emotional connection with her devoted husband, the "Knight of the Feather." She would be less needy from Al's perspective, and therefore less the fragile, vulnerable woman that Al fell in love with. In a real sense, Al needs a woman who needs him—and hence Al needs Anita's phobia almost as much as she does. Often without realizing it, he encourages her fear by his solicitous words and actions. In the current psycho-speak, Al is Anita's phobic enabler.

PHOBIC FEAR AS AN EMOTIONAL UPPER

In addition to its social value, fear taken PRN—that is, "when needed"—can serve as a morning cup of coffee or afternoon Red Bull or Coca-Cola to stimulate us. We have each developed adrenalin boosters that make us feel more awake, alive, and eager. Exercise fulfills that function for many people. Those who prefer vicarious exercise sit on the edge of their stadium seats or on their couches to cheer on their favorite sports teams. Some venturous souls seek out heightened danger experiences to get their juices going—extreme skiing (or *any* skiing for some of us), skydiving, auto racing, triathlon competitions, and other somewhat daring activities. In all these cases, our physical systems are stressed (in terms of pulse, blood pressure, breathing rate, and so forth) for a period, only to be followed by the "ah" response of relaxation, recovery, and return to physical stasis. We learn by experience to endure the more uncomfortable aspects of thrill experiences (whether in physical form, such as a churning stomach, or in emotional form, such as anxiety over possible harm) for the dividend of release from those feelings and the "endorphin high" that accompanies and lasts in the afterglow of high-stimulation experiences. A variety of drugs, including amphetamines, ecstasy, cocaine, and others are also used to produce physical and emotional stimulation.

Whether consciously or subconsciously, some people have learned to use their phobias as daily (and sometimes hourly or moment-to-moment) stimuli to produce heightened adrenalin states. We have seen in an earlier example (recall Wendy and Walter) how scary movies—and, by extension, Stephen King novels and even some of Shakespeare's more gruesome tragedies—are perennially popular for their ability to stir strong feelings and bring the "ah" response of eventual relaxation and recovery. Aristotle called this the *catharsis* (literally, in Greek, the "flushing") response, where hidden emotions of fear and insecurity become projected onto a dramatic protagonist, then eventually exorcised as that hero or heroine meets his or her fate.

Well managed, a phobia for some people becomes a personal psychic drama (a mental videotape of sorts) that can be run and rerun to arouse the fear response and the release/relaxation feelings that follow. Victor, for example, is said by others to "suffer" from agoraphobia. Over the years he has become more and more housebound. The prospect of vacation travel terrifies Victor. A simple trip to the grocery store is a major challenge for him. His wife and remaining friends (his illness has cost him many friendships) pity Victor and what they see as his self-imprisonment.

But consider Victor's own description of his difficulties:

> I don't really see what the fuss is about. I'm basically a shy person who doesn't like to go out much. So what? I'm perfectly happy reading a book, watching TV, or working at one of my hobbies at home. Not everyone is cut out to travel or run around town all day. My wife keeps trying to get me to see a doctor, but I wish she would just accept me as I am. I'm a happy person as long as I do things my way and don't get outside my comfort zone.

Just to be clear about his situation, Victor's "comfort zone" includes only the square footage of his home. The walk down his driveway to the mailbox is distinctly outside his comfort zone, as Victor explains:

> I do go outside each day to get the mail—and I admit that I get a bit shaky toward the end of the driveway. I feel

myself start to sweat and my heart starts to palpitate. Sometimes I feel light-headed and I need to sit down at the curb before making my way back to the house. But once I'm back inside I settle down and feel okay again within a few minutes.

Victor's daily routine of getting "a bit shaky"—that is, pushing himself purposely into a heightened adrenalin state associated with fear—sets the stage for feeling "okay again" once he has reentered his comfort zone. In fact, Victor has defined good physical and emotional feelings as the opposite of what he feels when he tries to walk down his own driveway to fetch the mail. He admits that on days when he does not go to get the mail he often feels "flat" and somewhat depressed. In effect, he is using his phobia much as another person may use a daily walk or jog—a period of stress that precedes and in fact makes possible the follow-up feelings of restored stasis and relative well-being.

PHOBIC FEAR AS A PERSONAL RITUAL

Consider one more case of a phobia used to "adrenalize" life experiences, in this case instilling a hormonal dose of instant courage. Evelyn, in her mid-50s, has developed over the past few years a phobic response associated with swallowing. She traces her problem to a choking episode at her 50th birthday party. She got a piece of sandwich stuck in her throat and spent several panicky moments in the bathroom desperately gasping for air. In the following days, she self-diagnosed the problem as a failure to chew her food properly and thereafter set out on a near-compulsive routine of chewing each bite completely, and then some, before allowing herself to swallow.

Evelyn's original swallowing episode had happened while she was eating at her table with friends and relatives. As is common with many phobias, it was the repetition of this general scene that seemed to bring back Evelyn's symptoms. When she was by herself she could eat quite comfortably (after thorough chewing, of course) and had little difficulty in swallowing. But social eating experiences were a different story, as Evelyn explains:

> I look around the table and I feel that the whole thing is going to happen again—that I will choke once and for all, that everyone at the table will be horrified, and that no one will be able to help me. I take a bite and chew it to

death, but it just won't go down. I try to will myself to
swallow, but I feel my throat muscles at the back of my
mouth physically lock up, almost as if I'm gagging. Of
course I try everything I can to prevent anyone at the table
from noticing my discomfort. If it gets intolerably bad, I
have to pretend to be coughing into my napkin while I
am actually spitting out the food in my mouth. This probably sounds very strange, but I find that if I can scare
myself—feel a little burst of panic—I can usually then go
on to swallow normally for several minutes or even the rest
of the meal.

Evelyn feels that she needs to "burn through" an adrenalized state of
fear to overcome her symptoms, however briefly. She has become used to a
particular phobic episode as a personal ritual that must precede normal
functioning. This phenomenon is well known to many people who experience "speaker's nerves" before or at the beginning of a public speech or
business presentation. As one speaker told us:

I feel terribly nervous for the first minute or so of my presentation, but then I begin to settle down and feel energized but not panic-stricken for the rest of the speech. I've
gotten to the point where I accept my nervousness as the
price I pay for a lively presentation. In fact, if I don't go
through my little period of panic, I worry that my speech
will be flat.

A similar use of phobias can be observed in many people who fear
flying. One patient explained the experience as follows:

I begin to get nervous a day or so before my flight, and my
fears build steadily as the time for take-off approaches. I
almost always reach the crescendo of my horrible feelings
of panic just when the plane is racing down the runway to
takeoff. I typically have a full-out panic attack at that time.
I feel like I have to get out of my seat and out of the plane.
I sweat like a pig and my heart rate goes nuts. But when
my panic attack subsides, usually after five or six minutes,
I feel so washed out and exhausted that the rest of the
flight usually goes okay for me. I sometimes even fall asleep.
I've never had two phobic attacks in a row. I can count on
at least a few hours of peace once I've had one.

The use of phobias to spark physical sensation is usually not a completely conscious willful act or choice ("I'm feeling a bit bored, so I think I'll turn on a phobia to get my system racing for a few minutes"). Instead, a phobic episode becomes habitual as "the way I get my symptoms to go away for a while."

PHOBIC FEAR AS AN EXIT STRATEGY

We all have life experiences that we dread—let's say, Thanksgiving dinner with the disapproving in-laws, an uncomfortable medical procedure, or a hot afternoon stuck in freeway traffic. And we have each probably developed coping strategies to help us through these events: "It's just one dinner a year and they get a kick out of seeing the kids." "The colonoscopy sounds awful, but my doctor says it's better than risking cancer." "I may as well turn on the radio and listen to a ball game. This traffic is going nowhere for a while." In short, we learn to talk ourselves into, through, or out of life's pinch points.

People with phobias have an additional arsenal of such exit strategies. These people often are the last to notice that their phobic episodes occur at suspiciously convenient times. Dan has been tabbed by his boss to take a business trip far from home. The day before the trip Dan experiences heart palpitations and breathlessness, with accompanying fears that send him to the emergency room. As in the past with Dan's spells, these symptoms upon examination can't be traced to any physical cause. But Dan nevertheless phones in sick with the explanation that he must miss the business trip while he undergoes a cardiac workup (his fourth in the last three years). Dan's phobic fears regarding his heart have become an unconscious exit strategy for career obligations he wants to avoid.

Another case in point: Barbara, 24, has a blind date coming up. It sounded like a fun idea last week when her roommate arranged it, but now that only a couple of hours remain before the guy is expected to show up to her door, Barbara is feeling familiar sensations of queasiness. She vividly remembers that at her 12th birthday party she had felt suddenly ill and had proceeded to vomit uncontrollably onto the party table and some of her guests.

In the years following, this episode, which Barbara recalls with everlasting embarrassment, has replayed itself a thousand times in her head, particularly at those moments when she finds herself socially "on stage," whether at a party, on a date, or in an interview situation. At these moments she felt as though she might vomit and, as she focuses on her fears of throwing up, her feelings of queasiness increased. Sometimes she has to leave the room either to get a drink of water or to sit quietly in the bathroom until the feeling subsides. At other times she makes up lame excuses about recent illness with food poisoning or stomach flu. She has experimented with antinausea medications without positive results.

The blind date knocks at the door. Barbara feels herself bathed in perspiration as she opens the door. "I'm so sorry," she says. "I have to cancel because I'm just not feeling well. I would have called but it came on so suddenly. I had Chinese food for lunch and I think it may be food poisoning." The young man graciously accepts her explanation and wishes her well—maybe a rain check for some other time. Barbara sighs with relief as he walks back to his car. Within a few minutes she is feeling fine again, and in fact orders a pizza for her own dinner.

What's going on here? From an outside view, Dan and Barbara are obviously using their phobias as excuses to avoid certain experiences. But consider the situation from their points of view. If we confronted them with the evidence that their symptoms tended to occur in suspicious connection with events they disliked, their response might be as follows: "My symptoms are real. I'm not imagining my heart beating fast (Dan) or horrible feelings of nausea (Barbara). You may think it's all in my head, but it's certainly not."

We could call this response the "neurotic equation":

Real Symptoms = Real Threats

Both Dan and Barbara believe that the absolute reality they feel regarding their symptoms automatically means that the threats associated with those symptoms are equally real. Put another way, the reality of what they feel convinces them of the reality of their perceived threats. For example, a woman with dog phobia does not say to herself: *That dog over there has no particular interest in me. The chances that I will be attacked are very slight.* (This version of the situation would, for most of us, accord with reality.) Instead, the woman runs a long-practiced phobic script that sounds something like this: *I'm feeling fear when I look at that dog. Therefore, it must be getting ready to attack me. Dogs sense fear. If I don't get out of here now that dog will probably start moving toward me. The more I'm afraid, the more the dog will become hostile toward me.* Notice here that the felt reality of the symptoms (panic and dread) get projected onto the perceived stimuli, in this case the dog. A vicious cycle ensues. The more the woman believes that the dog will harm her, the more acute her symptoms of panic and dread become. The more acute her symptoms, the more the woman attributes her fears to the dog.

Breaking the neurotic equation involves inserting a "does not equal" sign:

Real Symptoms ≠ Real Threats

At some point, the woman in the previous case must learn to say to herself: *I am feeling panic and dread, but those symptoms have nothing to do with the dog across the street. My symptoms will gradually decrease the more I see the dog as just a dog, not as a potential monster pursuing me. If the dog does begin to chase me, I have several ways I can get away from it.*

Some individuals, including rock climbers and crocodile hunters, learn to break the neurotic equation in reverse: they admit the reality of the threats before them (a 1,000-foot drop or a 12-foot crocodile) but do not let those very real threats lead automatically to the real symptoms of paralyzing fear that would beset most of us.

A HEALTHY RESPECT FOR THE FEAR RESPONSE

This book is dedicated to the lessening or complete dissolution of phobic feelings that interrupt life activities and spoil otherwise joyful and productive experiences. But extinguishing phobias does not mean getting rid of the fear response itself.

Our ability to experience fear, respond to fear, and remember fear has helped to ensure our survival from our earliest years. After a somewhat traumatic fall, a young child will learn not to crawl too near the edge of the bed. Touching the proverbial hot stove leaves a lasting (and often physical) reminder not to repeat that experience. Being scratched by a cat quickly convinces us not to hold the cat so tightly; being stung by a bee keeps us from touching the hive.

The most powerful of our fear responses is the often discussed "fight or flight" reaction, a physical and emotional syndrome programmed for trigger-quick firing within our deepest and oldest brain and related hormonal systems. Physiologists interpret this strong fear response to the early necessity in human prehistory to literally fight or flee in the face of mortal threat. When a saber-toothed tiger with lunch on its mind came menacingly toward a caveman, that ancestor relied on the fight or flight response to perform at least four immediate readiness routines to aid survival:

1. The heart beats faster and breathing increases, with heightened blood pressure, to ensure the flow of oxygenated blood to vital organs for the sake of strength in physical struggle or escape.

2. Perspiration cools the body to make possible maximum exertion without overheating.

3. A degree of nausea and/or diarrhea evacuates the digestive tract so that the body's resources can be devoted to higher priority survival measures.

4. The visual, auditory, and olfactory senses go to full sensitivity, with eyes darting about to assess the immediate environment (the familiar "rabbit eyes" seen in speakers under the influence of speaker's nerves) and the ears attuned to even the slightest sounds around us.

Not all sudden pains or surprises awaken the full might of the fight or flight response. By adulthood, our list of "burns" from learned fears is long indeed. What we define as safe behavior for ourselves and for others is, in fact, the path that remains after we have blocked off as dead ends the alternate paths that lead to pain and associated fears. Of course, day-to-day sanity requires that we do not call all of these formative fears to consciousness. They are "latent" in the sense that they guide our actions and choices but do not take center stage in what we think about from moment to moment.

But if "fear is our friend" as a general rule, what goes wrong in cases of phobia? For reasons we will explore in depth with illustrative cases, we sometimes attach grossly exaggerated emotional and physical reactions to particular fear experiences. Those who experience a fear of broken glass, for example, don't merely step around a broken bottle on the sidewalk (a normal response borne of experiencing or seeing a cut from glass shards), but instead react with a prolonged physical and emotional storm of aversion, with frightening images of glass piercing their flesh, blood flowing uncontrollably, and splinters of glass entering the bloodstream on the way to vital organs.

This exaggerated response to something that deserves a degree of caution (broken glass) is in itself frightening and often becomes a secondary stimulus to sustained phobia. Not only do severe fear responses feel uncomfortable, as hearts race, stomachs turn, and perspiration covers our bodies, but social discomfort amplifies our feelings of threat and embarrassment.

Others notice our struggle with fear symptoms and ask, "Is everything all right? Do you want me to call 911?" Because our fear response is so exaggerated, given the actual stimulus, we usually can't or don't want to try to explain our phobic response. It's difficult to say even to friends that "whenever I happen upon broken glass in my path I experience waves of panic that make it almost impossible for me to keep walking."

IMMEDIATE FEARS VS. REMEMBERED FEARS

Phobias would be of much less consequence in our lives if they reared their painful heads only when specific stimuli were present. For example, a person who fears clowns would avoid phobic suffering simply by staying away from clowns.

But thanks to our species' powerful faculty of imagination, we are able to "scare ourselves" without being in the presence of the feared object or experience. Images of the fear stimuli interrupt our quiet moments and haunt our dreams. The hint of circus-like music on television can bring clowns to mind, and with them irrational feelings of dread and fright to those who fear clowns. At the extreme edge of phobia, we may begin to fear listening to music at all, for fear that some sounds (a calliope, for example) may awaken our fears.

Remembered fears become all the more potent once we define ourselves as a person suffering from one or more phobias. After all, we each spend a significant portion of the day thinking about ourselves—who we are, what we want, and what others think of us. Those who conceive of themselves as athletes spend enormous amounts of time thinking about their weight, training schedules, eating habits, and physical prowess. Those who conceive of themselves as actors or actresses think about their dramatic opportunities, character motivation, emotional range, and attractive appearance.

Similarly, those who have defined themselves primarily by their phobias play these fears over and over in their minds. They wake up wondering if they will experience phobic suffering during the day. They spend the hours of the day trying to avoid phobic stimuli or recovering from encounters with phobic stimuli. They exert enormous amounts of energy in blaming themselves or others (Mom and Dad are popular targets) for their vulnerability to phobias. They return again and again in their mental and emotional life to memories of a recent or long-past phobic experience. Some phobic sufferers report thinking about their phobia dozens of times per day, as in the case of the claustrophobic individual who evaluated every space he occupied during the day according to its likelihood to "cause" feelings of smothering and imprisonment.

By such mental gymnastics, we replicate the original power of a phobic experience into hundreds of cloned stand-in experiences, so that daily life becomes a carnival fun house (though not so fun) with mirror-like reflections and distortions of our phobia(s). We see our fears everywhere we turn. We get used to scaring ourselves in ways large and small by the potential for, memory of, or hints associated with our central fears. For example, if we have an insect phobia, we check and recheck our domestic environment until we have assured ourselves that it is free of insects. Before going out, we play through the likelihood of encountering insects on our walk through the park (where a cloud of insects might suddenly buzz out at us), a ride in a cab (where an insect might fly in through the window and enter our clothing), or sitting on furniture in a lobby or waiting room (where hidden insects may crawl out to sting us). The fact that these things rarely happen (if ever) to us does not dissuade us from the need to busy our minds with insect checking. We get into our routine so thoroughly that we begin to forget what life was like before we had insects to think about.

The net result of such phobic influence on our daily lives is hydra-headed. In some cases, it yields chronic fatigue, as we waste adrenalin bursts on dozens or hundreds of mini-scares of our own imagining during the day. In other cases, it leads to distraction and an inability to think clearly and consistently about our work and personal tasks. Relationships inevitably suffer as others notice our self-obsession, withdrawal from social interaction, and general (and usually unexplained) timidity with regard to life experiences that bring fun and excitement to our friends. We seem to be "somewhere else," and in fact are in another mental place where the cross talk from phobic "what if's" and "watch out's" occupies our attention.

MIGRATING PHOBIAS

Many physicians, psychologists, and psychiatrists have noticed and written about the almost maddening phenomenon of phobias that migrate from one item or organ of obsession to another. In the case of hypochondria (an exaggerated focus and anxiety over one's physical health), a person's phobia may first present itself as constant worry over one organ—let's say, the heart. Alvin takes his pulse 20 or 30 times a day to make sure he is within the normal range for his age and activity level (as described to him by the Internet, of course). He calls his physician frequently about fleeting chest and arm pains. He lies down immediately upon feeling any "extra beats" (extra systoles) in his heart rhythm, to which he has become hyperattuned to the point that he can feel his heart beating in his fingertips, throat, and elsewhere at will.

Although Alvin's physician suspects that his cardiac symptoms, such as they are, have their locus more in Alvin's head than his chest, the doctor nevertheless performs due diligence by putting Alvin through a cardiac workup. After a month of tests and several thousands of dollars in fees, Alvin concludes that there is nothing wrong with his heart and that most people experience extra heartbeats from time to time. Alvin thanks his doctor profusely for helping to banish his heart fears.

Three months later, however, Alvin was back at his doctor with re-newed fears, this time focused on his kidneys. He had seen a television special on kidney failure, kidney dialysis, and kidney replacement. His occasional backaches, Alvin told his doctor, were clearly indicative of kidney failure. He had been drinking 12 glasses of water a day and taking tablets from his health food store in an effort to "purify" his kidneys and prevent stones. Again, Alvin's doctor cooperated by ordering a battery of tests to rule out various forms of kidney disease. Alvin once more was assured of his general level of good health and, more specifically, the healthiness of his kidneys.

Within a matter of weeks, Alvin had returned to his physician, this time with vague complaints about early-morning "jerkiness" in his muscles, particularly when he raised his hand to his shoulder in a bicep-flexing motion. Alvin suspected multiple sclerosis and, he confessed to his doctor, had been worrying himself sick about who would care for him in the final stages of his illness.

The process of ruling out illness after illness for people with migrating phobias is expensive, endless, and unproductive. People who want one or more dominating fears will find them in spite of all medical evidence to the contrary. With the help of his physician and follow-up sessions with a psychologist, Alvin was finally able to assess in a somewhat objective way his apparent *need* for phobias of one kind or another. Only when this underlying psychological state was addressed could Alvin free himself from an organ-by-organ, disease-by-disease series of obsessive fears.

THE NEED FOR PHOBIAS

As we have seen, the need for phobias can stem from an individual's attempts to be more socially sympathizable, from his or her deep-seated wish to escape from certain life experiences, and from the desire—conscious or subconscious—to "adrenalize" life by recurring pricks of fear.

In addition, some people need phobias to fill the void of a joyless, purposeless existence. Thoreau pointed to his aspect of the human condition in his famous dictum that "most men live lives of quiet desperation." The phobic response, for all the suffering it inflicts on the individual and those around him or her, has the effect of *thematizing* life—that is, making life *about something*. In Alvin's case, a relatively flat, uneventful, and generally unsatisfying life has been transformed by hypochondria into a life with issues—battles to be fought, mysteries to be investigated, challenges to be met. Phobic health concerns have given Alvin people to need (primarily doctors, nurses, and lab techs) and profound matters of life and death (his own) to think about. He can now read Thomas Mann's *The Magic Mountain* and feel a bond of empathy with the protagonist who gradually chooses illness as a way of life to stay in step with those around him.

Freeing Alvin from his hypochondria will prove exceedingly difficult so long as it is the raison d'etre of his existence. Simply desensitizing him, for example, to the beat of his heart will leave a psychological vacuum that he will quickly fill with phobic worries about other organs and illnesses. To move beyond hypochondriacal phobias, Alvin will have to discover another, more healthful theme and motive for his life. In short, he will have to substitute something that brings him deep joy for the things that now arouse deep fears. This process, usually beyond the scope of a primary doctor–patient relationship, will involve Alvin's commitment to honesty about what is missing in his life and his wholehearted resolve to pursue joy, by his definition, rather than run from fear.

As Alvin reviews his past several years of health phobias, he notices one period of about three months when he was relatively free from fear after slipping on an icy sidewalk and breaking his arm. During the time he was having his arm x-rayed and then set in a cast, and while it knit, he experienced few phobic symptoms. After all, he had his arm to think about. It gave him a regular reason to check in with his doctor and proved to be a useful topic of conversation with friends and acquaintances. Once his arm was out of the cast, however, Alvin's phobic symptoms and worries began to recur.

The realization that his phobias could be set aside by other, more pressing needs and feelings gave Alvin important insights that led to his eventual recovery. He made a list of activities that he sincerely enjoyed (as opposed to activities he was supposed to enjoy). From that list, he prioritized five enjoyable activities to which he would give his head and heart over a period of three months. He resolved not to let his phobias keep him from pursuing these activities. He wanted to find out once and for all if his pursuit of joys could substitute for his apparent and long-unadmitted need for fears. Alvin's list was highly eclectic: he wanted to build a harpsichord; complete an orchid greenhouse in his backyard; take a cruise to Alaska; forge a closer relationship with his two nieces, whom he adored; and lose 15 pounds. Any one of these items, Alvin told his doctor, would bring him deep satisfaction. He hadn't given time and attention to their achievement, he explained, because he hadn't been feeling well (due to his hypochondria) and couldn't find the time in the midst of frequent medical appointments.

But once Alvin found himself elbow-deep in tiny wooden parts from a do-it-yourself harpsichord kit, he was a pig in clover, unable and unwilling to turn aside from the pleasure of his work to worry about his spleen, appendix, or duodenum. He had found his own personal recovery route from hypochondria and phobias in general not in a "mind over matter" philosophy, but instead in realizing (and practicing) the insight that when we are eager to do something, we don't let much hold us back. We throw off what the poet William Blake called "the mind-forged manacles" and get on with the joy of living.

PHOBIAS AS SELF-PUNISHMENT

Many people believe they have done something wrong and therefore deserve punishment in some form as their present reality or future fate. Their "sins" can range from disappointing their parents or not measuring up to a stellar brother or sister, to causing a divorce or failing in school or business. Instead of facing up to their situation and moving ahead with the life they want to live, these people "beat themselves up" by thinking negative, self-critical thoughts about their looks, personalities, activities, and friendships.

Part of this self-flagellation can involve phobias—particularly fears that are future-oriented.

The guilty person, convinced that punishment is on its way, obsesses over the monsters that hide just around the next corner. They perceive themselves as bad people to whom, inevitably, bad things will happen. For example, 25-year-old Jill labors under the impression that, to please her parents, she should have done better in college and should now have a much more prestigious, good-paying job (like her older sister Janice has). She feels that she lives under a dark cloud that dooms all new beginnings and activities in her life to eventual failure. She pictures herself as desperately treading water to avoid being washed away entirely.

In this context, Jill has noticed that her teenage phobia about heights (acrophobia) has become much worse in recent months. She had to quit her executive assistant position at an insurance company because her office was on the 40th floor of a downtown high-rise. Even though her desk was far from any windows, she nevertheless felt vaguely dizzy and nauseous at the thought of being more than 400 feet off the ground. Especially after the 9/11 tragedy, her thoughts ran often to what she would do and how she would feel if a fire broke out in the building. She fantasized in a nightmarish way about being herded toward a broken window and having to jump into a fireman's net far below. In her imagination she heard herself screaming "I can't! I can't!" as the flames crept closer to her. Jill dreaded going to work and never accepted her friends' invitations to use the open-air garden at the top of the building for lunch.

Jill has negotiated with herself to feel reasonably comfortable up to the fifth floor of any building, so long as she can take the stairs to get there. She allows herself to attend job-seeking interviews at any office up to that height. On two occasions she has been offered positions, but had to decline them because they were in offices above the fifth floor. She has thought about going back to school for a master's degree, but the classroom buildings at the only college in town are high-rises with crowded elevators and huge glass windows everywhere.

Jill says she worries that "the walls are starting to close in on me." On some days, she can't depend on herself to feel comfortable even up to the fifth floor. She worries what her life will be like when she can't be two or three floors above the ground, even while shopping at the mall, without feeling her dreaded symptoms of light-headedness, nausea, and high anxiety. Jill feels that things are getting worse and holds out little hope that therapy (which she can't afford anyway) will help her.

Jill doesn't discuss her fear of heights with friends. Like her college grades and her job track record to date, Jill feels her fear of heights is one more thing to be ashamed of and to hide. She sees herself in a closed circle of frustration: her unhappiness fosters her fears, and her fears, in turn, guarantee her continued unhappiness.

Of the many dysfunctions Jill could settle upon to be unkind to herself—anorexia nervosa, drug abuse, sexual promiscuity, and so forth—she has subconsciously self-selected a phobia custom-made for her needs. It applies directly to the areas of her life about which she feels most guilty. First, it keeps her from achieving her professional goals (and thereby gaining, at least in her mind, increased esteem from her parents). Second, it neatly prevents her from returning to school to improve her academic record (and thereby erase her guilt over a mediocre college record). Finally, it isolates her from many of her friends and excludes her from many of their activities. In effect, Jill has invented a day-in, day-out punishment that fits the guilt she feels.

Jill's escape from her made-to-order acrophobia must begin by cutting herself some slack in the short term and learning to love herself in the long term. Probably no single insight, New Year's resolution, pill, or therapy session will suddenly make Jill's acrophobia disappear. More likely, she will have to go through a transition period during which she concentrates on "doing what's comfortable for me and makes me happy." She won't pursue job opportunities that reinforce her inadequacies and, in effect, punish her for her perceived failures. She will do whatever she must to find a comfortable job where she feels valued, no matter how that position is evaluated by her parents or sister. Once she grows into new life patterns relatively free of self-punishment, she can probably look forward to the gradual alleviation of acrophobic symptoms. At some future point, she will ask herself not "Why did heights make me panic?" (her earlier way of perceiving her dilemma), but instead "Why did I need to panic in high places?" (her new perception based on recognition of her own role in selecting and sustaining her phobia).

THE ART OF DESENSITIZATION

Psychologists have long observed the "wear-down" effect of the same stimuli repeated over and over. Let's take a person who suffers from fear of spiders (arachnophobia). When he is shown a picture of a spider, he may react with revulsion and feelings of incipient panic. Those feelings may be present for the second, third, and fourth picture shown to him as well. But by the 10th or 20th picture (especially if accompanied by reassuring language, calming music, or accompanying pleasurable imagery), the person's panicky reactions tend to dull, eventually to the point of boredom. In this case, boredom with formerly high-voltage stimuli is much to be desired.

The phobic person will ideally conclude from such exercises that a stimuli (the image of a spider) does not necessarily or automatically produce uncomfortable feelings—that he can "stand" such stimuli without giving in to anxious feelings. This insight by itself can be inspiriting for the phobia sufferer and can contribute to the eventual extinguishment of the phobia.

In reality, most people with phobias experience a rebound effect between desensitization sessions. In other words, they begin Session Two of desensitization with anxiety levels not much reduced from the levels experienced at the beginning of Session One. Their habitual phobic responses, learned perhaps over a period of years, have a perverse way of reasserting themselves and partially canceling out the progress of earlier work. But in gradual steps ("two forward, one back"), the emotionally freighted images of the feared object(s) build up an inoculation against phobic response.

As described earlier in this chapter, some forms of phobia have their roots in depression, post-traumatic stress disorder, obsessive-compulsive disorder, and complicated low self-worth issues. Although the symptoms associated with phobias can be relieved by desensitization therapies, many medical practitioners find that the sufferer's unresolved psychological problems and pressures bring back phobic symptoms after a period of time, often in the guise of new fears and anxious obsessions. The goal of complete therapy, therefore, is to resolve the underlying causes of a phobia as well as its surface symptoms.

A COMMON CASE OF DESENSITIZATION: THE FEAR OF FLYING

We can generalize about the symptoms of phobias without denying that individuals experience phobias, just like grief and loss, in very different ways. Let's take one of the most common phobias—the fear of flying— and follow it in one person's case from its first occurrence to the height of its often agonizing symptoms:

Brent, a 30-year-old Realtor in Columbus, Ohio, hadn't flown since college days. He made his living within a 100-mile radius from home and was able to drive to his business appointments. But when his company was bought out by a large Chicago corporation, Brent was asked to fly to that city to interview as manager of Columbus operations. On the Tuesday of his flight, Brent showed three homes to clients in the morning and then raced to the airport to make his 1 p.m. flight. He flopped into his seat on a smallish, crowded plane. The air circulation vents hadn't been turned on and the cabin of the plane was warm and stuffy. Brent wiped perspiration from his brow and loosened his tie. The woman next to him buried her nose in a magazine.

"Ladies and gentlemen," the captain intoned over a scratchy sound system, "we have a gate hold for the next 15 minutes or so. Sorry for this inconvenience, but we will make up time once we're in the air. We'll get the electrical cables hooked up again in a few minutes and get the cabin cooled off. Thanks for your patience."

Brent sighed audibly and shifted in his narrow seat. He worried about showing up late for his interview in Chicago. He took off his sports coat and noticed sweat circles on his previously impeccable shirt. Brent pulled at his collar and tried to cool off.

A strange sensation passed across his chest and shoulders—certainly not a pain, but more like what he had felt once before when his swinging car stopped at the top of the Ferris wheel.

Brent felt his breath coming in shorter gasps and took off his seat belt to remove any constriction from his waist. He felt the woman next to him look sideways to see what was the matter.

The sensation came again, more powerfully. Brent felt an overwhelming need to get off the plane. He half rose in his seat, but quickly sat down again when he saw that the gangway had pulled back and that the fuselage door had been sealed.

Brent closed his eyes and tried to breathe deeply. He felt his heart racing faster, the sensation of panic now rising from his chest into his neck and face. He knew he was sweating profusely and hoped the people around him didn't notice.

Suddenly the plane jerked forward and, within a minute, was blasting at full speed down the runway. Brent, fully at the panic stage, felt that he could not get enough air and forced himself to take fast, irregular gasps through his mouth. His eyes were clenched shut and his fingers dug into the armrests. The plane lurched upward and powered at a steep angle into the air. Brent fought off the strong need to rip off his seat belt and somehow try to get off the plane. His head told him he was stuck on the plane, but other voices inside were screaming for him to do something, anything, to get free of his seat.

He opened his eyes and saw the red pulse of his soaring blood pressure at the edges of his vision. He felt like he was looking out of a darkening tunnel. His head felt like it was going to explode. His heart palpitated with a hard thump, then another before racing on in a more regular rhythm. *I'm having a heart attack,* Brent thought to himself and immediately called to mind the horror of a cardiac problem at 30,000 feet without hope of help. He felt suddenly nauseous and dizzy. The cabin swam around him and he clenched his eyes shut again in an attempt to hold it together.

Suffice it to say that Brent survived the one-hour flight from Columbus to Chicago. But he got off the plane deeply shaken by his experience and physically limp from the ordeal. To his wife's confusion, he took a bus home from Chicago and, like John Madden and other flight phobics, has not flown since.

Brent did not pass out, as some panic sufferers (notably Tony Soprano on HBO) do. Nor did Brent experience stabbing chest pains, often confused with angina. But Brent looks back upon his "airplane meltdown" as the worst single hour of his life. He associates his symptoms exclusively with flying and does not expect to experience such panic again so long as he avoids airplanes.

In Chapter 3 and elsewhere, we will investigate in detail the forms of cognitive behavioral therapy (CBT) that can be used to desensitize Brent to his anxiety symptoms associated with flying. For now, we can simply outline that course of treatment. Brent would first undergo a thorough medical evaluation to make sure his symptoms indeed stem from phobia and not from one of many physical conditions. Then Brent would participate with his physician and/or psychiatrist or psychologist in one or more in-depth conversations about his problems. Based on this inquiry, Brent may be treated with an anxiety-relieving drug at first to ease his first efforts at confronting his fear of flying. In guided steps, Brent would probably read about the admirable safety record of modern airlines and the extraordinary steps taken by these companies to ensure that every plane is fit to fly. In stages, Brent would learn to sit comfortably in a plane on the ground, graduating to a plane rolling down the runway, and eventually to short flights. With the steady support of his doctors, Brent would spend considerable time in and around airplanes to confront and finally dispel his anxieties.

Chapter 3

HOW CAN I RECOVER FROM MY PHOBIAS?

This chapter answers five questions:

1. How does healing begin for phobias and related emotional illnesses?
2. What medical means can support recovery from phobias?
3. What is the integrative approach to ending phobias?
4. How does the mind–body connection generate the fear response?
5. What is meant by a chemical imbalance in the brain and how can it be corrected?

So far we have described phobias as mental and emotional sticking points—distorted versions of selected aspects of reality (such as a barking dog or a creepy-crawly spider).

Fortunately, we are not stuck with these painful and disruptive perspectives. We have the ability to change our thoughts and beliefs. Our minds are capable of deleting outdated or dysfunctional "programs" and replacing them with corrected and updated versions. We can grow, gain perspective, and learn new tools to deal with our fears.

In order for these important changes to happen, both the emotional and rational mind must participate. To aid such participation, modern medicine has shed a bright light onto the neurological causes and treatment of anxiety and phobic disorders. For some patients, it makes as much sense to fight a phobia without medical treatment as it does for an army to engage in a modern conflict armed with only bows and arrows.

In the many cases discussed so far, we have seen that phobias learned through emotional experience are not easily influenced by input from the rational mind. You may strongly *feel* that you are in imminent danger while all the time *thinking* you are safe. For example, a person in the throes of a phobic attack during an airline flight may be able to tell you that air travel is significantly less dangerous than auto travel. Information available to the rational mind will often not be enough to stop the physiologic symptoms of anxiety, including elevated heart rate, nausea, dizziness, shortness of breath, chest pain, a sense of impending doom, and so on. This disconnect between our rational powers and our emotional nature is especially clear when a person goes through a relationship breakup. Rationalizing that the relationship was going nowhere and not "meant to be" does nothing for the emotional hurt and suffering. How we feel cannot easily be thought away.

Overcoming a phobia requires that we change our thoughts and beliefs using both our rational and emotional minds. An important first step is to examine the rationality of our fear and to determine accurately the true level of danger that the fear poses. Yet, as discussed, the emotional mind does not often change by logical persuasion alone. Intelligence alone usually will not suffice in overcoming a phobia with deep roots in the emotional mind. The most powerful unlearning of a phobia occurs through the same experiential, emotional mode by which it was first learned. This process of unlearning means that direct (and sometimes coached) exposure to a phobia, even if it temporarily causes anxiety to increase, is an emotional experience that allows the mind to truly believe that the feared catastrophe will not happen. The more this correction of a distorted version of reality sinks in on a conscious and subconscious level, the more your physical and psychological experience of fear will diminish.

As self-confidence rises, you will learn to react differently to the situation that previously brought on phobic reactions. Experience teaches your emotional mind in a way that facts and figures cannot. As the poet Keats wrote, "The axioms of philosophy are not axioms until they are proved on the pulses." Avoidance of the feared stimulus leaves open our doubts about "what will happen" when the next confrontation occurs. Only by gradually exposing ourselves to the feared stimulus, albeit in a controlled and supported way, can we make significant progress in the recovery process. Just as a patient with a pulled muscle is advised to stretch gently to the point of discomfort but not pain, so a phobic sufferer must enter a process of desensitization through exposure. This process is accomplished in small increments that combine bearable discomfort with feelings of progress and achievement. No phobic sufferer has to metaphorically or literally leap into a snake pit or wallow in worms (a la TV's *Fear Factor*) to attack a phobia successfully.

MEDICAL SUPPORT IN THE DESENSITIZATION PROCESS

Some people will require some level of medical sedation to even *begin* to get close to the feared situation. Common treatment involves small doses of short-term antianxiety medications used at the beginning to get through the initial stages of the process. We call this "medical desensitization." Similarly, for those struggling with anxiety and mood disorders, effective medical intervention is now available. Untreated, these underlying conditions distort our perspective on desensitization and destabilize the necessary neurological environment for healing and recovery to take place. Through thoughtful selection of the proper medication, today's physicians and psychiatrists can chemically balance the nervous system more effectively than ever before. Many anxiety conditions, for example, can be stabilized virtually overnight, with full control possible within a few weeks. Such treatment includes a regimen of therapy aimed at gaining insight into our dysfunctional patterns of thought and to identify our stressors. Only when anxiety disorders and stress are under control are we able to make progress with the experiential methods of desensitization.

For all the virtues and advantages of pharmaceuticals, it is important to recognize that medication can be misused as an avoidance strategy. Instead of thinking through our life patterns and confronting our fears, we pop a pill. For this reason, many psychotherapists feel that medication can slow the recovery process. There is some evidence that those who use only cognitive behavioral therapy, or CBT (therapy that does not involve medication), have lower rates of relapse than those who used CBT with medications.

Therefore, except in the case of medical desensitization, where anxiolytic drugs (see Chapter 7) are used only during the initial stages of exposure therapy and then quickly withdrawn, the medical treatment of phobias is not generally recommended. However, anxiety and mood disorders—which up to 80 percent of phobic patients live with in addition to their phobia—should be treated if they are significant obstacles to recovery. We are not open to new learning by any modality when our mind and body are racked by waves of acute anxiety, panic attacks, or severe depression.

AN INTEGRATIVE APPROACH TO RECOVERY

In short, the development of a phobia relies upon an underlying hypersensitivity and often a chemical instability of the nervous system. A variety of methods have been discovered and tested in the course of modern medicine and psychotherapy that contribute to this process of reduced sensitivity and stabilization. What we believe to be the best of these tools are gathered and explained in the remainder of this book. Several approaches are provided so you can pick and choose the tools that reflect your beliefs and sensibilities. Among these tools you will find advice for a healthy lifestyle; psychotherapeutic approaches of cognitive behavioral therapy and psychoanalysis; exposure therapy; stress management; appropriate medical treatments; mind–body techniques of acupuncture, massage, aromatherapy, music, meditation, biofeedback, and the relaxation response; herbal and supplemental remedies; and an enlightened spiritual perspective.

Unlocking the nature of your particular phobia and attacking it at the source will likely require some combination of these tools. Historically, the treatment of phobias has lacked an integrative approach that recognizes the value of several therapeutic tools used in meaningful combination or sequence. Too many people with emotional disorders, including phobias, continue to feel that their responsibility to their recovery ends with taking a pill. Many spend years going from doctor to doctor in hopes of finding the dispenser of the "right" pill. In fact, no medication alone has been shown to be the sole factor in recovering emotional health. Only a broad, integrative program that involves your complete commitment can turn around a thought, a disorder, or a life. We will show you how to construct such a program customized to your specific needs. To assist you, we have designed the Anxiety Toolbox Program (available online at *www.anxietytoolbox.com*) to guide you through the elements of the recovery process in a step-by-step manner. But only your perseverance and dedication can bring about the desired transformation. The expression "no pain, no gain" could appropriately be rephrased as "no comfort without some discomfort" when it comes to the hard work of changing phobic beliefs and habits.

THE PHYSIOLOGY OF FEAR

We all try to avoid phobias when possible because they trigger strong and unpleasant physical symptoms. These arise from the body's alarm system, which is designed to tell us when we are in true danger and to quickly teach us a firm, memorable lesson that will protect us in the future. In phobias and anxiety disorders, these high-intensity alarms go off when there is no true threat. The painful lessons of "don't go there," "avoid that animal," "stay away from needles," and so forth are learned nonetheless in the emotional mind. We tend to avoid exposure to the feared object or situation thereafter, no matter how nonsensical our behavior may seem to others and even to ourselves.

One of the main problems in the development of phobias is the misinterpretation of the symptom attacks caused by our anxiety alarm response. Unfortunately, many phobia symptoms such as shortness of breath, numbness and tingling, chest pain, and dizziness are also common in serious health events like heart attacks and strokes. Patients have every reason to seek medical care, often at ERs, when these symptoms strike. Although this immediate recourse to medical evaluation is understandable, it often creates a huge expense and heavy utilization of medical services at all levels. In the real world of defensive medicine where litigation lurks around the corner, each case must be taken seriously and worked up to first rule out a true catastrophic possibility. When an anxiety attack is the diagnosis, the physician should then clearly explain what happened and why. Lacking such explanations, the anxious patient will likely be back at the ER within a few weeks seeking answers and reassurance regarding his or her symptoms.

ACCURATE KNOWLEDGE AS A FIRST STEP TOWARD CONTROL

Understanding the physiology of the fear response makes us less likely to misinterpret our symptoms, thereby preventing the development of phobic avoidance behavior and stopping our anxiety from spiraling out of control. This chapter will explain what exactly happens in your body when you experience phobic anxiety. A clear understanding of *what* your body is doing and *why* may have prevented your first phobic attack, particularly if you were also able to control your apprehensions about what others were thinking about you at that moment.

THE MIND–BODY CONNECTION

We already know intuitively that how we feel physically affects our emotions, and how we feel emotionally affects our physical sense of well-being.

We are not only what we eat, but also what we think, feel, and believe. In fact, the influence of mental and emotional states on physical well-being has been one of the dominant areas of medical research in recent decades. Dr. Herbert Benson of Harvard Medical School first described the "relaxation response" after studying the physiologic changes in meditating Tibetan monks. He showed how, through exercises of the mind, they could control such body functions as heart rate, temperature, and sweating. As lie detector technology reveals, changes in levels of emotional stress can dramatically influence physical factors. We are now in a position to use information on the mind–body connection to carry out more successful healing strategies, including ways to overcome phobias.

EVENTS IN THE BRAIN

Although they may be felt in the chest and elsewhere, phobic anxiety reactions begin in the brain. They affect the brain from the highest cortical centers and temporal lobes to the deeper, more primitive structures in the limbic system, basal ganglia, brain stem, and spinal cord. Once aroused by phobic alarms, the brain sends urgent electrochemical messages through the central nervous system, which in turn communicates with every cell and organ in the body directly or indirectly through peripheral nerves and chemical/hormonal messengers in the bloodstream. This immensely complex system of communication goes a bit haywire if a chemical imbalance occurs in the brain, with implications for false messaging to the rest of the body. A phobic episode is often the net effect of such a chemical imbalance.

If biology class wasn't your thing, the following information on brain chemistry may seem a bit too schoolish. Nevertheless, many phobic sufferers find themselves somewhat relieved to learn that physical factors within the brain (often inherited) account for many aspects of their phobic symptoms. Imagine for a moment the unnecessary frustration in blaming pain from a broken arm on a failure of courage, personality, or character. In a similar vein, many phobic sufferers have been blaming themselves for feelings that have a real physical cause. Therefore, we hope you will take time to at least get the basic idea of how the brain and central nervous system process alarm signals. In this section, we offer a level of detail about brain chemistry that your physician or other health professional probably cannot take the time to give you. In short, here's your chance to glimpse "how it all works" within the sophisticated systems of the body.

Monoamine Balance

For four decades, the main theory to explain the biochemical basis of emotional dysfunction has been the "monoamine hypothesis." According to this theory, anxiety, panic and depression result from imbalances of one or more of three biochemicals known as monoamines, namely serotonin, dopamine, and norepinephrine. These are the neurotransmitters that allow and facilitate communication from one neuron to the next, and one nerve pathway to the next. When there is a prolonged deficiency in the amount of monoamine compounds, the receptors on the head of the receiving neuron become more plentiful in a process called "up-regulation." This phenomenon correlates directly with the onset of depression and anxiety. Because it takes weeks for up-regulation to occur, it also takes weeks for normalizing "down-regulation" to occur with treatment. This explains why it takes several weeks for medical treatment to be effective. Popular SSRI (selective serotonin reuptake inhibitor) medications (Paxil, Prozac, Zoloft, Celexa, Luvox, Lexapro) improve serotonin levels. Tricyclics and MAO (monoamine oxidase) inhibitors increase all three monoamines. Drugs that stimulate release of monoamines from the neuron or prevent reuptake by the receiving neuron include the newer drugs Effexor (serotonin and norepinephrine), Wellbutrin (dopamine and norepinephrine), and Serzone (serotonin and norepinephrine).

SEROTONIN BALANCE

Serotonin is produced in the neurons from the amino acid tryptophan. It is released into the synaptic clefts by a nerve impulse, and then destroyed by monoamine oxidase after it does its job. This brain neurotransmitter is perhaps the key player in anxiety conditions. All the anxiety disorders, including obsessive-compulsive disorder (OCD), panic disorder (PD), post-traumatic stress disorder (PTSD), and generalized anxiety disorder (GAD) have been successfully treated by medications designed to enhance serotonine in the brain. Cell bodies of the serotonin system reside in the median and dorsal raphe nuclei of the brain stem. Projections go to the frontal cortex (mood); the temporal lobes (panic/anxiety); the deep limbic and basal ganglia (mood and anxiety conditions); the hypothalamus (appetite and eating behavior); the brain stem (sleep center that regulates slow-wave restorative sleep); the spinal cord (orgasm and ejaculation); and the gastrointestinal system (cramps, diarrhea, constipation, and nausea). This latter connection explains why serotonin deficiency can cause irritable bowel syndrome (IBS).

As the serotonin system is weakened by stress, the anxiety response is more easily triggered. Deficiencies can stimulate the sympathetic ("fight or flight") response, while normal levels inhibit this system and promote parasympathetic discharge (with calming effects on the nervous system). Many conditions lead to serotonin deficiency in the brain: chronic fatigue, chronic pain, hormonal changes, insomnia, and emotional stress. Serotonin neurons have a restraining effect on the periaqueductal gray area, the area of the brain stem involved in the panic response. The presynaptic neuron has a reuptake pump to salvage the serotonin and pump it back into the cell to stop neuronal communication. It is controlled by the 5HT1A presynaptic receptor. The 5HT1D presynaptic receptor blocks the release of serotonin when stimulated, and the alpha-2 receptor blocks the release of serotonin when norepinephrine binds to it. Drugs that inhibit these receptors allow an increase in serotonin release into the synapses, and have been found to be effective in the treatment of depression, OCD, GAD, PD, PTSD, as well as social phobia, drug/alcohol dependency, chronic pain, seasonal affective disorder, and the eating disorder bulimia nervosa.

NOREPINEPHRINE BALANCE

The neurons of this system are located in the locus ceruleus of the brain stem. These neurons make norepinephrine (NE) from the amino acid tyrosine. Through the action of three different enzymes, tyrosine is first converted to dopamine, and then to NE.

The locus ceruleus is responsible for determining whether our attention is focused on the external environment or internal environment. Anxiety is a state where we are acutely aware of how we feel internally in our minds and bodies; there is little ability to enjoy the present moment, experiencing things outside ourselves. The locus ceruleus is the region of the mammalian brain that receives incoming information from all areas of the body, thereby monitoring the internal and external environments of the body. In turn, the locus ceruleus is wired to many areas within the brain known to be involved in the fear and anxiety response, including the amygdala (fear); the limbic system; the hippocampus and hypothalamus (emotions, energy, psychomotor retardation/agitation); frontal cortex (mood); prefrontal cortex (attention); the spinal cord (sympathetic activation to the bladder and heart); and the cerebellum (tremors). Hyperactivity in the NE system in the locus ceruleus is involved in the development of panic disorder. Electrical stimulation of this area in monkeys causes a fear response, while destruction reduces fear. The NE system in humans completes its neurodevelopment by the early 20s and degenerates with age. This may explain why the onset of panic disorder frequently occurs in the early 20s, and seems to "burn out" as a person ages.

DOPAMINE BALANCE

Dopamine, also synthesized in the neuron from tyrosine, is cleaned up from the synapses by the same chemicals—MAO and COMT (catechol-0-methyl transferase)—that remove norepinephrine from the synapses. Presynaptic dopamine neurons have a reuptake pump and a host of receptors, the most studied of which is the D-2 receptor. Drugs that stimulate the D-2 receptor are helpful in Parkinson's disease. Drugs that block the D-2 receptor slow down the transmission of dopamine nerve impulses, which helps schizophrenia, a disease caused by overactivity of the dopamine neurons. Proper dopamine balance is essential for normal functioning of the basal ganglia. Attention, pleasure/reward and motivation depend on dopamine balance.

The Benzodiazepine/ Gamma-Aminobutyric Acid Neuronal System (GABA)

This system is an extensive network of linked neurons capable of modulating and suppressing neuronal excitement throughout the brain. When drugs known as benzodiazepines bind to the GABA receptors, the GABA neurons activate, thereby inhibiting the anxiety and panic response and causing muscle relaxation. Valium was the first benzodiazepine, originally invented as a muscle relaxant. Benzodiazepines are also useful in treating seizures and for the short-term treatment of insomnia. Newer hypnotic agents such as Ambien, Sonata, and the drug Gabitril bind reversibly to GABA receptors.

Neurokinins

These peptide neurotransmitters are strings of 11 amino acids (unlike the monoamine neurotransmitters, which have one). One neurokin called "substance-P" has been studied in the brain and the peripheral body. In the body, it acts as a mediator of neurogenic pain, released during times of injury and inflammation. In the brain, it seems to be responsible for our perception of pain in the amygdala. This may explain why those with poorly controlled anxiety complain of an increase in physical pain. Drugs that block substance-P appear to have an ability to decrease pain and anxiety in some individuals.

Melatonin and the Pineal Gland

Like serotonin, melatonin helps the nervous system adapt to a changing environment with the least amount of stress. Melatonin and serotonin inhibit the sympathetic nervous system (fight or flight response) and stimulate the parasympathetic system, which is associated with calming. Melatonin increases GABA, another important neurochemical in controlling anxiety. Melatonin helps us adapt to basic environmental rhythms, such as night and day. As night falls, melatonin increases and becomes a key player in signaling the start of various mental and physical restorative processes. It also accounts for much of the body's temperature rhythm, allowing the nighttime temperature drop required for sleep. Unlike serotonin, melatonin passes through the blood–brain barrier, and can therefore be taken directly as a supplement.

Most of the brain's melatonin is generated in the pineal gland through the conversion of serotonin. The pineal gland has a particularly elaborate blood vessel system, and serves as a key modulator of the entire neurohormonal system. It is the gearshift that allows us to adapt to changing environmental conditions. Because the pineal gland is light-sensitive due to connections with the optic nerves, it allows the brain to perceive the time of day.

Melatonin deficiency has been linked to depressed mood, sleep disruption, disturbed body rhythms, agitation, increased anxiety, and higher body temperature.

Prostaglandins and Anxiety

Originally discovered in the prostate gland more than 60 years ago, these hormones are made from only one source: essential fatty acids. Helping control the release of serotonin, prostaglandins are at the center of research in understanding depression and anxiety as well as a wide range of general medical conditions, including arthritis, multiple sclerosis, and even AIDS.

You can get essential fatty acids through dietary sources or supplements. The body makes two kinds of prostaglandins, sometimes labeled "good" and "bad." In reality, both kinds are necessary for survival.

The "good" prostaglandins promote immune response, reduce inflammation (helping arthritis), inhibit cell proliferation (protecting against cancer), inhibit platelet aggregation (preventing blood clots), and promote blood vessel dilation (protecting against heart disease). The "bad" prostaglandin hormones balance these effects (for example, allowing your blood to clot when it needs to, etc.). The balance of these hormones depends on stress, age, illness, and the presence of a key essential fatty acid eicosapentaenoic acid (EPA), which is found in high concentrations in fish oil.

What we eat affects the good-to-bad ratio of prostaglandins. Simple carbohydrates such as sugar increase insulin, which promotes the bad prostaglandins. Good prostaglandins (PGE1s) have been shown to be associated with an elevated mood (thought to cause the initial elation of alcohol), and bad prostaglandins (PGE2s) increase with anxiety, anger, or hostility.

The Deep Limbic System

The deep limbic system is at the center of the brain. Only about the size of a walnut, it is critical for human emotion and behavior. It is an "older" part of the mammalian brain, setting mammals apart from the reptiles, a class of animals that behaves in a more predictable way dictated by the brainstem. This is why a dog is apparently more emotional than an alligator. The dog forms limbic bonds through physical contact such as licking and smelling. Human beings also store emotional memories, such as the smell of something (or someone) we love, the taste of a food we are passionate about, a voice we trust (or fear), and so forth. The deep limbic system adds the emotional desire, passion, and drive to our organizational, problem-solving, and rational cerebral cortex. It is in this part of the brain that our phobic emotional memories are stored and triggered when we are confronted by a phobic stimulus.

When the deep limbic system is quiet and calm, there is generally a positive and hopeful state of mind. When it is overactive and heated up, negativity takes over. Hyperactivity in the deep limbic system directly correlates with negative emotions. This was demonstrated consistently in SPECT scan studies by Dr. Daniel Amen, M.D., a clinical neuroscientist and specialist in behavioral medicine and brain imaging techniques. SPECT stands for "single photon emission computerized tomography," a nuclear medicine study that "looks" directly at cerebral blood flow and indirectly at brain activity through level of metabolism. The deep limbic system sets the emotional tone of the body, stores emotional memories, promotes bonding, modulates libido, processes sense of smell, controls appetite and sleep, tags events as internally important, and sets the emotional tone of the mind. Problems in this system cause moodiness, irritability, depression, negative thinking, negative perspective, appetite and sleep problems, social isolation, decreased or increased sexual responsiveness, and problems with motivation ("I just can't get started").

Women, on average, have larger limbic systems than men, giving women the advantage of being more expressive of and "in touch" with their emotions. Typically, women are better able to bond and connect with others, helping to explain why they are the primary caretakers of children in all societies on Earth. But women are also more susceptible to depression, especially at times of hormonal change. Women attempt suicide three times more often than men (although men are three times more successful because they use more violent means). Men are more likely to be disconnected from others due to less limbic bonding.

The deep limbic area is "wired" by nerve connections directly to the prefrontal cortex, the supervisory part of the brain that takes up to about age 21 to fully develop. When the deep limbic system is activated, emotions take control, while the more rational prefrontal cortex is inhibited. Often, the more emotional you become, the less rational and "in control" you are.

The Amygdala and Basal Ganglia

The amygdala and basal ganglia deserve special mention due to their central role in anxiety. The central nucleus of the amygdala is where learning processes relevant to fear and anxiety occur. In turn, its neurons are strongly interconnected with the hypothalamus and the brain stem regions, which are responsible for triggering the physical symptoms of anxiety and panic. When the amygdala neurochemical N-methyl-D-aspartate (NMDA) is blocked, the acquisition of conditioned fear responses is also blocked. The basal ganglia are a set of large structures located toward the center of the brain surrounding the deep limbic system. They are involved in the integration of feelings, thoughts, and movement. They set the body's "idle speed," or anxiety level. The functioning of this area of the brain accounts for why you jump when you're excited, tremble when you're nervous, or get tongue-tied when you're angry. It decides how easily you startle. If there is too much input, as in an accident or other stressful situation, they tend to "lock up." People who already have overactive basal ganglia due to an anxiety disorder are more likely to be overwhelmed by stressful situations, freezing up in action and thought. Those with attention deficit disorder (ADD) have been found to be underactive in the basal ganglia. In this case, the stressful situation moves them to action. They are often able to react without fear to a stressful situation, and they are frequently the first on the scene of an accident. Underactive basal ganglia are associated with low motivation and energy, while overactivity causes anxiety, tension, increased awareness, and heightened fear. Many highly motivated individuals show increased activity in this area, which may be the key to their success. The drug Ritalin increases dopamine release in the basal ganglia, helping motivation, mental focus, and follow-through. Cocaine powerfully increases dopamine in the basal ganglia, and, interestingly, so does love.

Problems in the basal ganglia are implicated in anxiety; panic; physical symptoms of anxiety (i.e., heart pounding, difficulty breathing, nausea, sweating, hot or cold flashes, dizziness, feeling faint, tension headaches, sore muscles, and hand tremors); low threshold of embarrassment; quick startle reaction; tendency to predict the worst; worry about what others think; fear of dying or doing something crazy; feeling off-balanced; shyness and timidity; pessimism; conflict avoidance; Tourette's syndrome (TS); muscle tension/soreness; tremors; fine motor problems; headaches; and low or excessive motivation. TS involves involuntary physical movements and noises such as coughing, puffing, blowing, barking, and sometimes swearing (coprolalia). It can be inherited through several genetic abnormalities found in the dopamine family of genes. Sixty percent of those with TS have ADD, and 50 percent have obsessive-compulsive disorder. All of these seem to have a similar connection through dysfunction in the basal ganglia.

Cognitive behavioral therapy and guided imagery are especially helpful in quieting overactive basal ganglia, as is deep breathing and meditation/self-hypnosis. Anger and stress management are also important in quieting the basal ganglia.

Emotional Molecules

Medical schools in the mid-1980s taught that the nervous system and the immune system operated relatively independently of one another. We have since discovered that nerves connect the immune system to the nervous system, which is directly wired to the brain. We have also found a host of neuropeptides—molecules that carry messages between the brain and every cell in the body, enabling them to be in constant communication with one another. The brain and endocrine system are also in constant communication through direct nerve channels and bloodstream-borne chemical messengers. As Candace Pert, Ph.D., author of *Molecules of Emotion: The Science Behind Mind–Body Medicine*, states: "The mind and the body are really inseparable. They're one."

The somatic dysfunctions caused by phobic anxiety attacks can be explained fully by this interconnection of the mind and body through the nervous system and chemical messengers. During the fight or flight response, the mind, under the influence of fear, sends neurological and chemical signals to the endocrine glands, the heart, gut, muscles, and blood vessels (i.e., the body) to react in predictable ways. These signals alter, redirect, and disrupt the normal regulatory functions of the body, causing a myriad of symptoms.

Valuable Information From EEG/PET/SPECT Scan Studies

Electroencephalogram (EEG) studies have shown that panic disorder is linked to an inherited trait of low-voltage alpha waves (the brain waves involved in the "relaxation response"). Alcoholics with anxiety are 10 times more likely than a normal control group to have low-voltage alpha waves. Depressed patients exhibit a reduction in alpha wave (REM) sleep time. Neuroimaging techniques such as positron-emission tomography (PET) and single photon emission computerized tomography (SPECT) scans show differences in brain structure, circulation, and metabolism between those with emotional illness and normal controls. These studies have shown that frontal, temporal, and limbic/hippocampal areas are activated in panic disorder patients. The amygdalocortical pathway is activated during fear conditioning. Depressed patients show activation of the deep limbic system.

The Sympathetic and Parasympathetic Nervous System

Fear can originate in the conscious, highly developed cortex of the brain, or the deeper, more primitive centers that control our emotional and subconscious awareness. In either case, the signals of fear reach the hypothalamus gland. The hypothalamus in the seat of the deep limbic system is a crucial brain structure in understanding the mind–body connection. It translates our emotional state into physical feelings of relaxation or tension. The front half of the hypothalamus sends calming signals to the body through the parasympathetic nervous system, while the back half sends stimulating fear signals via the sympathetic nervous system. It is the sympathetic system that triggers the fight or flight response when faced with a threat. A combination of parasympathetic inhibition decreasing vagus nerve input and increasing sympathetic activation causes increased heart rate, breathing rate, and blood pressure; the hands and feet go cool and the pupils dilate (presumably to see better).

The hypothalamus also makes control hormones that tell the pituitary gland which endocrine glands it should activate. By producing ACTH-releasing hormone at the time of stress, it causes the pituitary to release ACTH, which then circulates through the bloodstream to the adrenal glands, causing them to release "stress hormones" such as adrenalin, noradrenalin, and cortisol. These hormones bind to receptor sites on cells, and can activate a variety of responses and symptoms, including tremors, sweats, a more forceful heartbeat, diarrhea, nausea, and hyperventilation with light-headedness. Beta-blockers are drugs that block the beta receptors where these hormones attach, thereby stopping these unpleasant symptoms.

SYMPATHETIC NERVOUS SYSTEM

Hypothalamic triggering of the sympathetic nervous system (SNS) activates a cascade of hormonal and neurological messages that flow throughout the body, exerting an effect on many different organs, systems, and functions of the body:

Cardiovascular: The heart rate increases and the amount of blood pumped out with each beat (stroke volume) increases. These factors result in an increase in the blood pressure to improve circulation. Blood flow is also redirected as involuntary smooth muscles that surround our arteries are stimulated to either relax or constrict. (Relaxation causes the artery to open up and allow more blood flow to the more vital tissues; constriction cuts back the circulation to less important areas.) The blood carries the necessary nutrients, especially oxygen and sugar, faster and in larger amounts to the big muscles of the arms and legs, and the heart, lungs, and brain. In contrast, blood flow decreases to the skin, hands, feet, kidneys, and digestive system during the fight or flight response. You may notice that your hands and feet go numb, tingle, or feel cold during anxiety attacks due to this aspect of SNS activation. Additionally, the blood coagulates faster to protect against excessive blood loss in case of injury. This combination of higher blood pressure and hypercoaguability may make some individuals more vulnerable to a stroke or heart attack during a period of anxiety.

The symptoms of a heart attack are common during hypothalamic triggering of the SNS, with 35 percent of those experiencing anxiety complaining of chest pain and heart palpitations (fast or irregular heart rhythm).

Pulmonary: Breathing becomes deeper and faster to supply more oxygen to the larger muscles that may be asked to fight or run. As we hyperventilate, we not only get more oxygen into the blood, we also blow off the carbon dioxide as we exhale, reducing the blood concentration of this gas. This imbalance in blood gases can also lead to dizziness, nausea, and numbness and tingling in the arms and legs.

Sweat Glands: Increased sweating is stimulated by the SNS, thereby helping the body to regulate its temperature. Some patients describe this phenomenon as "breaking out in a cold sweat."

Central Nervous System: The mind goes on high alert, as all senses become heightened and we are capable of focusing intensely on the present danger (or, in phobic situations, what we erroneously perceive as the present danger). This full alert can be seen on a brain wave machine (electroencephalogram) as a rapid firing of beta brain waves. Emotions of anger and/or fear arise from the basal ganglia and amygdala centers deep in the brain. At this point we may sense an overwhelming sense of doom. Many people having an anxiety attack for the first time, especially if the attack is severe, truly feel they are dying.

Behavior: During SNS activation caused by a phobia, we will usually either fight or flee. Imagine someone with a phobia of bees. One lone honeybee may set off an angry and aggressive flurry of flailing arms and legs in an attempt to kill the creature or motivate a person to jump into the nearest body of water. The reaction of paralysis is also possible, the fear so powerful that the person cannot move, scream, or react. He or she will often say of the experience: "I was so scared I couldn't move or speak. I was paralyzed with fear."

PARASYMPATHETIC NERVOUS SYSTEM

The functioning of the parasympathetic nervous system (PNS) is required to reverse all the physiological events previously described. The heart rate is slowed down through parasympathetic vagus nerve stimulation, also reducing stroke volume and blood pressure. Blood flow returns to the hands and feet as smooth muscle contraction in the peripheral arteries begins to relax. Breathing slows, restoring a normal balance of oxygen and carbon dioxide in the blood, and sweating subsides as our temperature drops back down to normal. In the mind, beta brain waves decrease as alpha brain waves amplify.

(One of the main goals of the Anxiety Toolbox in Chapter 9 is to teach practical strategies for stimulating the parasympathetic nervous system to counteract, or "balance," a hyperactive sympathetic nervous system.)

Chapter 4

Understanding Phobic Anxiety in New Ways

This chapter answers five questions:

1. What are the positive values of fear and "good anxiety"?
2. How can emotional false alarms be distinguished from helpful fears?
3. What are 10 core truths about anxiety that are often forgotten or obscured during phobic suffering?
4. In what sense do we sometimes love the very phobias that plague us?
5. Why does society seem to enjoy watching fearful reactions and phobic suffering on television?

The main purpose of this chapter is to challenge your perceptions, beliefs, and attitudes about phobias and anxiety in general. After all, anxiety symptoms triggered by your phobia are probably what led you to this book and your decision to fight your way back to a joyful life unencumbered by unnecessary fears.

By understanding anxiety—even to the point of appreciating its contributions to health and safety—we can place phobic fears in proper perspective and reduce their hold over us. Consider, first, that we human beings, like all animals, develop fear responses for *protection*. The fight or flight response involves the involuntary nervous system and causes a powerful and instant reaction to a perceived threat. Even if the threat turns out to be a false alarm, as in the case of a friend jumping out from behind a door and yelling "boo," our sympathetic nervous system has been activated before we have a chance to countermand it. Even after we have concluded that no danger is at hand, we may feel a pounding heart and other fear symptoms for many minutes. This leap-before-you-look response on the part of the body is healthy and adaptive. After all, in our evolutionary history it was always better to be safe by reacting quickly rather than thinking too long and ending up the meal of a saber-toothed tiger.

Another useful behavior unfairly given poor press these days is *avoidance*, which occurs in anticipation of danger. We typically think of avoidance as a bad thing, as in the case of a spouse who won't discuss a pressing problem ("You're just avoiding the situation"). In a larger perspective, avoidance serves the function of steering us clear of situations that might result in personal harm. We may choose to avoid the automated bank teller at 2 a.m. in a bad neighborhood. In this case, our anxiety and avoidance tendencies may preserve our well-being.

It is useful to think of both the good and bad aspects of anxiety or, more generally, the functional and dysfunctional uses of fear. In dysfunctional anxiety, we pay attention to false alarms, reacting with fear to situations that pose no real threat. Avoidance behaviors then follow as we abandon rationality to shun future contact with the dreaded stimulus. In this way, one dysfunction leads to follow-on dysfunctions, causing more limitations, blocked paths, and missed opportunities in our lives. We may take a further step and attach especially powerful fear responses to a particular thing, experience, or situation—in which case we have saddled ourselves with a phobia. (Because such phobias often arise from an underlying anxiety condition, this chapter will briefly discuss the various types of anxiety disorders, along with examples of the dysfunctional phobias and other emotional problems one might expect to experience with each of these conditions.)

GIVING CREDIT TO GOOD ANXIETY

Good anxiety helps us in many ways beyond its contribution to our physical protection. George W. Brown, a renowned clinical psychologist, has described anxiety as a fear of future loss. This fear motivates us to study for the final exam, work extra hard to make our business a success, and cherish our relationships lest we lose them. Many experts feel that emotional stress, manifest in the form of anxiety, grief, and depression, serves as the driving forces that shape our identity and psychological development.

It can also be argued that anxiety is a social glue of sorts that holds us together. Why, for example, do we get married? Of course there is physical attraction, but just as potent in our stroll to the altar are our emotional needs. In large part these needs arise out of anxiety—the fear of spending life alone, the fear of missing out on having children, and the fear of not having a spouse who understands and supports us. Anxiety makes a baby cry out for his parents when he wakes up from a bad dream and wants to be held. Anxiety over possible social alienation steers a willful teenager back to her social group to apologize for some unkindness. Some believe that such emotional forces also allow a higher level of enlightenment and are necessary for spiritual growth. Anxiety has been described as an inner voice telling us our lives are not in balance—that we have neglected our emotional or spiritual health. In 1844, Danish theologian and philosopher Soren Kierkegaard wrote in *The Concept of Dread* that we fear our own freedom most of all: "Consciousness of the future expresses itself as dread. But the future does not exist, it is nothing. And yet, unlike the past, which is solid and unchangeable, the future, *my* future, must still be created by me, in my freedom. I create my future through my every choice and decision. I must even create *myself* in the future. Dread is the fear of the awesome responsibility of self-creation. It is a fear of freedom." Or in Sartre's words, "I await myself in the future. Anguish is the fear of not finding myself there."

Faced with our inner fears, we become acutely aware that we stand alone as unique and free individuals, personally responsible for what our future will become. (In Chapter 9 we will turn specifically to a discussion of lifestyle choices that, in essence, create our future and largely define who we are.)

In short, accepting full responsibility for your future inevitably includes accepting our worries about what will happen in that future. Anxiety should not be banished as the prodigal child of emotions. It speaks messages to us that are painful at times to hear and feel, but are nevertheless vital to our individual growth.

DISTINGUISHING FALSE ALARMS FROM USEFUL FEARS

It is easy to understand how a false anxiety alarm can happen. Take, for example, the interesting case of Denise, a 47-year-old woman who found herself under a great deal of stress. She had just received the final papers ending her 19-year marriage. Her teenage son was in legal trouble on drug possession charges, and her car needed repairs that were not in the budget. In addition, she was skipping her periods and having problems with sleep, which her doctor said was common with stress and perimenopausal hormone changes. Overwhelmed and exhausted, she went to the bank to open a new account in her name. While filling out the forms, on the section that requested information on marital status, Denise suddenly felt dizzy, nauseated, and thought her pounding heart would beat right out of her chest. Not knowing if she would faint or throw up, Denise quickly excused herself from the bank representative and walked briskly to her car in the parking lot. Before getting there, she threw up into the bushes. Acting as though her keys had dropped on the ground, she was able to disguise what had really happened.

Denise experienced a false alarm. Her fear response system had fired off, triggering the sympathetic nervous system and all the usual symptoms that are the mind and body's normal reaction. There was really no threat to her life or health, but this obvious truth did not stop the physical symptoms from happening. It is useful to note that Denise's nervous system was already on high alert, just looking for trouble. This hypersensitivity can be expected to happen when we are under undue stress, sleep deprived, and having hormonal upheavals all at the same time. We call this a state of heightened arousal of the nervous system, just ripe for developing a phobia.

But something else is needed for a phobia to really take over. We must either misinterpret what has happened or misperceive the reaction of others to our attack. Denise thought for a moment that her heart palpitations and dizziness could be the sign of a heart attack. At the time she thought about having the bank call 911. Then an image came to her of paramedics ripping her shirt open while the other customers standing in line at the bank watched in horror. Another image, just as revolting, involved throwing up full force on the bank employee. She immediately feared the disgust of both acquaintances and strangers nearby. Better to escape to the car! The misinterpretations and misperceptions that accompanied this experience is what turned the *false* alarm into a *learned* alarm, or phobia. Because she feared another attack could happen at any time, Denise began avoiding public places where she might be humiliated by vomiting, fainting, or having someone insist on calling the paramedics. She was not afraid of the panic attack, but of humiliating herself in public. She began avoiding the bank, the grocery store, the mall—until eventually she really only felt comfortable at home. She had not had any attacks in these other locations, but learned to fear them just the same.

Through this process of fearing her anxiety symptoms as they might unexpectedly occur in public places, Denise developed agoraphobia. Öhmann and Mineka (2001) make the point that humans, because of our sophisticated nervous system, do not have a preprogrammed fear response. We have an adaptive system that can learn new responses. Because of this capability, we can learn to fear an external situation such as going to the bank or the mall, or an internal sensation such as a rapid heartbeat or dizziness. According to Barlow and Graske (1994), when a false alarm occurs in a situation where escape is difficult, the intensity of the anxiety is heightened. This amplification results in strong emotional learning. In the bank, Denise felt somewhat trapped. How could she get away without drawing attention to herself? What would the teller think if she walked out in the middle of her account application? Yet staying would open up the possibility of scrutiny by others and inevitable embarrassment.

Following her jolting experience in the bank, Denise would feel uncomfortable whenever she was in a public place that prevented ready escape.

Is Denise doomed to feel comfortable only in her home (the "housebound" dilemma that results for many agoraphobics)? Fortunately, we have the ability to change our learned alarms. For Denise, the first requirement was to quiet the high arousal level of her nervous system. This stage of therapy was accomplished through treatment of the hormone deficiency and improving her sleep cycles with a nonaddictive sedative. She also chose to learn how to amplify her calming alpha brain waves through a series of five biofeedback sessions, started a regular exercise program, and reduced the carbohydrates in her diet.

When she began feeling stronger, she began exposure therapy, where she stayed for increasing periods of time in situations that were uncomfortable for her. She eventually learned that it was unlikely that an attack would occur, and if it did, people would really not think less of her or be disgusted by her symptoms. As her life stressors improved, Denise was able to leave her agoraphobia behind for good.

Core Truths About Anxiety

Those who have experienced high anxiety states for a prolonged period as part of their daily living come to identify themselves as "anxious" people. Anxiety, in other words, becomes one of the main traits by which they describe their core natures and personalities. To break the hold of phobias and anxiety, such people must be challenged to think and feel differently about themselves, often with the help of a therapist. Such changes often involve giving up snippets of "health information" gleaned from TV and the Internet. Even when such bits of information are true, they may have no direct applicability to a person's own case. The myths you grew up with as well as your own misinterpretations about the scrutiny of others and your own misperceptions about internal sensations must be countered regularly by reality and truth.

Here are the common truths that should be learned, memorized, and taken to heart. If these dictums seem counter to your usual ways of thinking about yourself and your struggles with phobias and anxiety, all the better—they are then direct challenges to the ways of thinking and feeling that so far have proven unproductive and painful for you.

Anxiety is an integral and natural part of the human experience. Anxiety is a necessary and useful emotional experience that allows adaptive, experiential learning and teaches us about our true self. We do not have to apologize for feeling anxiety, nor is the absence of anxiety and fear our goal in this admittedly precarious life on Earth. However, we should learn to keep anxiety in its place. We can learn the lessons it has to teach without letting it dominate our daily thinking and feeling.

Anxiety is not out to kill you. Anxiety is a valuable response designed to protect and motivate us, not to destroy or damage us. It can only damage us if we give it more attention than it deserves. It would be folly to say that no one has ever died of an anxiety attack. Anxiety, like anger, is a strong emotion that causes strong physical responses. A person with a weak heart or untreated blood pressure could experience a fatal event. On the other hand, death during or immediately after an anxiety attack is statistically quite rare. The medical and psychological literature on phobias and anxiety contains thousands of documented cases of anxiety attacks that led to no physical damage whatsoever. A healthy person has nothing to fear from anxiety, other than the disruptive lifestyle effects of fear itself.

Anxiety and panic attacks have natural limits. Even if you do nothing, your nervous parasympathetic nervous system will eventually counteract the anxiety attack, as it is designed to. You won't go crazy or find yourself in a straitjacket in an asylum (as the movies like to depict emotionally distraught people). Even if you actually faint or vomit, this physical action will usually abort the attack very quickly.

Understand that anxiety is a common fear. Rather than fearing anxiety, use it to discover *what* you fear. Identification of your fear is a crucial step in stopping the fear from terrorizing your nervous system. Usually the fear is very specific. Your assignment is to define it clearly, perhaps with the help of a therapist.

Anxiety involves the threat of future loss. Of course, those who have suffered previous loss are prone to worry about future loss. That is why those with depression and grief over the past often develop worry and anxiety as their primary emotions in dealing with the future. But living behind ourselves in the past with depression and ahead of ourselves in the future with anxiety prevents us from living joyfully in the present moment. And the present is what matters most. It is the only moment in which we can act to influence our future. We literally cannot reach back into the past to change things or reach forward into the future to guarantee anything there. Unless we are willing to let go of unnecessary future worries and past regrets, we cannot change our lives for the better today or grow in a meaningful direction.

The object of your fear and anxiety is not the problem. Don't blame the phobic stimulus for your anxiety condition. The buzzing bee, barking dog, jerky escalator, or hypodermic needle is not exerting some magic influence to "force" you to feel anxiety. Your discomfort lies in how you interpret and perceive the situation or object of your anxiety. Your goal should be to fix perception and attitudes, not fix the world.

The more you try to control anxiety, the more it will control you. The paradox of anxiety is that you must accept your anxiety to neutralize and render it powerless. Ignore it and it will go away; focus on it and it will become more acute. A pertinent case in point is the difficulty some people experience in swallowing pills. When the person focuses on the pill in their mouth, it feels like a walnut-size object that just won't go down. But when the person forgets for a moment about the pill (perhaps by looking in a mirror, with the inevitable effect of diverting interest to their face), the pill slides down as easily as all the other millions of morsels they have swallowed in their lifetime.

Anxiety takes what you give it. The more of your life you give over to anxiety, the more it will take. The more you let anxiety determine your choices and make your decisions, the more limited your choices and decisions will become. Cling to your right to experience joy and pleasure in your life.

Anxiety attacks will last as long as you allow them to. Fear is fuel to the fire of anxiety. The more you fear an attack and let yourself get worked up over it, the more it will spread and magnify in your consciousness and your life options. Self-hypnosis, biofeedback, and breathing exercises (as taught in the Anxiety Toolbox in Chapter 9) work by turning the mind's hypervigilant state of attention to a state of blithe disregard for false signals of alarm.

Avoidance ensures that your anxiety problem will get worse. You can't overcome a fear by avoiding it. The less you know about your fear, the further away you are from conquering it. Avoiding exposure increases apprehension and decreases confidence. Although medication can help stabilize the nervous system, you will still need to build your self-confidence through the experience of exposure. The person who deals with a fear of flying by the total avoidance of flying obviously has not resolved his or her phobia.

PHOBIAS WE LOVE TO HATE

Consider the following scenario. While cleaning pieces of wood out of his garage, Jack gets a sliver in his finger. Because this slight injury hurts, especially when Jack presses on his finger, we would expect him to remove the sliver as soon as possible. But Jack delays. He tells his wife that he wants to show the slivered finger to their kids when they arrive home from school. In fact, Jack decides, he will keep the sliver in his finger so he can show his buddies on the bowling team tonight.

"But doesn't it hurt?" inquires his wife.

"A bit," Jack replies, "but only when I press on it."

After dinner, Jack excuses himself from the task of doing dishes—"My sliver," he explains. Nor can he wheel the trash can out to the curb without discomfort. But later that evening, he is able to bowl quite well after showing his sliver to one and all on the team.

"How do you bowl with a sliver in your finger?" the team captain asks Jack.

"I just play through the pain," Jack responds, to the admiration of his teammates.

When Jack arrives home, his wife devotedly asks how his finger is feeling. Jack smiles bravely and tells his wife that he will be strong for her and the kids. The next day Jack manages to get to work, but can't drive a coworker to the airport because the steering wheel might press too painfully on his finger.

At this point, you are probably ready to shout, "Why don't you simply pull out the sliver?" The answer should be obvious. Jack has learned to value his sliver for all it can do for him. In a word, he *loves* his sliver. Notice that the sliver lets Jack slide out of distasteful tasks, such as doing the dishes and taking out the trash. The sliver gives Jack something special to show to others and brings, in return, the doting attention of his concerned wife. Finally, the sliver lets Jack play the hero at home and work as he courageously battles the physical curse that has befallen him.

Some people (but certainly not all) who suffer from phobias have befriended these mischievous irritations. Fear of flying, for all its inconveniences, brings such people an unspoken and sometimes subconscious reason for not traveling across country to visit with the in-laws, or, in a business context, to spend weeks away from the family on work trips. Fear of dogs may carry with it a certain pleasure as friends scurry to hide their pets in preparation for a visit from the "Special One." At the bridge table, dog phobia becomes a reliable and riveting topic of conversation as the Special One holds forth on her quite dramatic symptoms—"my heart feels like it is going to burst," "I begin to perspire all over"—when face to face with Lassie. Alice has her son who is a doctor, Virginia has her trust fund, and Wilma has her phobia. We all have to have *something*—and we go to extraordinary lengths to take care of what we have.

In the same way that phobias begin to define what's special about us as a magnet for the attention of others, phobias also provide a handy excuse for avoiding unpleasant or otherwise challenging tasks and experiences. Richard, now 45, has cherished his phobia of spiders since his teenage years. Thanks to his phobia, Richard has managed to avoid all gardening and yard care, all outdoor home maintenance, and a good portion of indoor cleanup and remodeling as well. The prospect of coming across a spider has prevented Richard over the years from taking his children on camping trips and traveling with his family to parts of the world where spiders are more common.

Although Richard complains about his spider phobia, he knows at some level that it is a not an unwelcomed guest in his psychological boardinghouse. On balance, Richard gets more from his spider phobia than he loses in terms of life convenience, ease, and enjoyment. As Nietzsche quipped of God, so with Richard and his phobia: if spider phobia didn't exist, Richard would have to invent it.

We could view Richard's situation as eccentric but inconsequential. What does it matter if he has fooled himself (and others) into the belief that he suffers from spider phobia, with all that it keeps him from doing? Sadly, the impact of phobias ripples out to families, friends, and coworkers. In Richard's case, his children missed out on camping trips "because Dad has his spider problem." The stressful and expensive responsibility for house and yard care falls on his wife "because Richard gets so upset." Business trips to rural locations become someone else's problem "because Richard won't go there." Depending on the phobia at hand, others who love the sufferer can themselves become victims of quite devastating theft—loss of emotional and sexual intimacy, loss of enjoyable recreation experiences, and loss of personal time—as the phobic person looks more and more for the support of others to cope with daily life. Making someone into an enabling crutch may bring tears of gratitude to the eyes of the phobic person, but usually without much recognition of the stress put on that crutch by the full weight of emotional reliance. Perhaps saddest of all, children learn many phobic responses and behaviors from their parents, and are themselves condemned to nervous attacks and limitations throughout their lives.

The proposition that we often love our phobias seems patently absurd to many phobia sufferers, as we might expect. After all, recognizing one's affection for phobic distress and its associated emotional manipulations means looking behind the curtain of the Great Oz to find the little man pulling the levers. Understanding the love process at work in some phobias forever changes our ability to believe in the reality and power of those phobias. Even in the midst of a panic attack due to fear of clowns, goldfish, flies, or whatever, we hear a nagging internal voice questioning whether we are in fact masking our real issues and aversions by a showy display of phobic camouflage.

Let's say, for example, that Julia, in her heart of hearts, fears death and the signs of aging that prefigure it. We will further assume that Julia can't or won't express these fears to those closest to her. She feels literally and figuratively trapped with her own intense feelings. She yearns for some kind of escape and release from her recurring thoughts of morbidity. On one particularly hectic day, she sprints to catch an elevator to her 30th-floor apartment, only to have it stop unexpectedly between floors halfway up the building. She finds herself utterly alone, trapped in a stalled elevator.

In spite of her best rational efforts, Julia feels huge adrenalin waves of panic rise from her stomach to her neck and face. She screams for rescue. Help comes within a matter of minutes, but her rescuers find a sobbing Julia huddled in a fetal position in a corner of the elevator. After months of therapy, she concludes that she "has claustrophobia," and must avoid enclosed spaces at least until such time as her ongoing desensitization therapy is successful.

What has been lost and what has been gained in the acquisition of this new phobia? Julia certainly recalls the elevator experience with terror ("cold sweats all over again," she says) and to that extent she has lost a portion of her inner peace and calm. But Julia also now knows how to avoid those feelings of panic and terror: simply avoid enclosed spaces such as elevators, underground transit cars, "submarine" amusement rides, her closet at home, and so forth. Her phobia has given her a new focal point for fearful feelings. Her earlier broad range of morbid thoughts and worries are now localized in one horrible, but ironically helpful, set of memories.

Julia's future course through life becomes an elaborate ballet of managing and protecting her feelings against a repeat of "the elevator experience." She "is doing better," she tells her friends, and measures her progress in terms of the number of hours, days, or months without "those" feelings. She accepts the idea that she may live with claustrophobic fears for the rest of her life and takes comfort in the fact that many people manage quite productive and happy lives in spite of claustrophobia. In a phobia-savvy society, she has very few embarrassing moments when she must act to avoid a flare-up of her phobia. Coworkers understand that she needs to take the stairs instead of the elevator. Friends know not to ask her to climb onto a crowded bus or subway.

In effect, Julia has put her major fears on hold (her fear of aging and death) while she teases herself with minor stand-in fears: the elevator experience. In the process, Julia is denying herself the opportunity to confront the deepest levels of her anxiety and perhaps break through to forms of confident, joyful living of which she cannot now conceive.

THE FEAR FACTOR OF PHOBIAS

Reality television has, for better or worse, been the most profitable new segment of network programming in this decade. Among the audience-attracting stars of this type of show are those such as *Fear Factor*, which features phobic or near-phobic individuals confronting their most piquant fears. For example, Alicia, who fears snakes, signs on with the producer for $1,000 and a trip to Los Angeles to let snakes crawl all over her bikini-clad body. John, who fears heights, allows himself to be strapped to the top wing of a biplane for aerial loop-the-loops for the camera.

At least three aspects of this social and psychological phenomenon are interesting. First, these phobic individuals demonstrate that, far from being embarrassed by their phobias, they are ready and willing to exhibit them for the enjoyment of others. This is an extreme form of the love-me/love-my-phobia use of fears by more average individuals in our culture. Second, television audiences give their time and television sponsors give millions of dollars to support this display of high anxiety. What exactly do people like to watch? As gruesome as it may sound, audiences enjoy watching participants squirm, shudder, and fight back nausea (sometimes unsuccessfully) as they eat worms, allow bees to swarm over their bodies, or tread water in the midst of a vast ocean without a boat in sight. The visible discomfort of program participants, often turning to outright panic, is apparently "fun" to watch because in the comfort of our living rooms we vicariously identify with what they are going through. We imaginatively toy with the idea of being in their situation.

Notice in this regard that television producers choose only the most universal phobias to exploit in their programs. Audiences aren't interested in watching Bill's anxiety over paper, let's say, as he is forced to walk through a room filled with crumbled newspapers. Such voyeurism would seem ghoulish to most of us, precisely because Bill's dilemma is so pathologically unusual. But when a phobia is generally shared by audience and participant alike—as in the case of fear of falling, fear of insects, and so forth—we don't feel that we are "picking on" a single sad, sick individual. Rather, we are watching one rather typical individual (to whom we may even ascribe bravery) going through what we ourselves would avoid like the plague.

We also enjoy watching in *Fear Factor*-like programs the character transition that engages us in all drama: we observe the rising suspense of the approaching fears, the climax of terror, and the eventual denouement as the individual at hand describes how he or she felt during the ordeal.

Importantly, the components contributing to the success of such programs also get played out in the daily lives of some phobic individuals. Television has no exclusive patent on using phobias to entertain others. Because phobic sufferers know that phobic displays (and associated talk about phobic feelings) have a certain degree of entertainment value for friends and acquaintances, these individuals don't hesitate to "go onstage" from time to time to act out their fears in front of others. (Some phobic individuals, in fact, confess that they seldom experience phobic reactions when they are alone—a telling confirmation of the hidden motive to use phobias as a social attraction.)

Here's the reaction of one phobic individual, Robert, when he confronted the possibility that, at a subconscious level, he was encouraging his own phobias by putting them onstage for the enjoyment of others: "When I began to seek treatment for my claustrophobia, I knew that I probably wasn't aware of some of its deep causes. After all, I was acting unreasonably in feeling claustrophobic in the first place. I had to assume that I would learn surprising things about myself that I couldn't figure out alone. But I never in a million years expected to face up to the idea that I was using my phobia to solicit a certain reaction from others. Now that I think back on my many claustrophobic episodes, they were almost all in the company of my wife or a close friend. The usual scenario was that I would begin feeling panicky, then I would confess my claustrophic problem (for the umpteenth time) to my wife or friend, who in turn would comfort me and help me either bear the situation ("talk me down") or physically remove myself from the place. It occurs to me that I may have married a woman who finds deep fulfillment in coming to the aid of a person in an emotional crisis ("he makes me feel needed"), and I may have sought out friends who feel the same thing. Basically, I am putting on a psychodrama that they have learned to anticipate and even enjoy. The cruel irony is that until this moment I didn't realize I was the actor and they probably didn't think of themselves as the participating and enabling coactors and audience."

In some cases, such realization brings release from the stranglehold of phobias. The new set of thoughts ("I'm doing my phobic thing to get something from others") can serve as a script that runs counter to, and tends to destroy, the threadbare "what-if" scripts that probably accompanied phobic thinking and feeling in the past. At the first impulse of phobic sensations, we start to accuse ourselves of giving in to narcissistic impulses, ignoble motives, and the manipulations of others.

Put more positively, we identify what we really want—in Robert's case, the caring response from his wife and friends—and find more productive, less personally painful ways of achieving that response. Robert eventually learns that he doesn't have to go through claustrophobic meltdowns to keep his wife and friends emotionally close to him.

Chapter 5

BECOMING FAMILIAR WITH DIFFERENT TYPES OF PHOBIAS

This chapter answers four questions:

1. What is agoraphobia and how does it sometimes lead to a "housebound" condition?
2. What are the main categories of specific phobias?
3. What is social phobia?
4. What is the prognosis for phobias left untreated?

So far we have seen by precept and example that phobias are exaggerated and irrational fear responses. Phobias can be broadly divided into three types: agoraphobia, specific or "simple" phobias, and social phobias. In the United States, the lifetime prevalence rate of phobias is about 13 percent. Collectively, these disorders are the most common forms of psychiatric illness, surpassing rates of mood disorders and substance abuse. Severity can range from mild and unobtrusive to severe, and can result in incapacity to work, travel, or interact with others. Death is uncommon, although suicide can occur in cases of severe agoraphobia, especially if associated with panic disorder. The occurrence of phobias appears equally distributed among races. All phobias cause similar physical symptoms because they all cause sympathetic nervous system activation, regardless of the object of the fear. Sympathetic activation results in a faster heart rate and higher blood pressure, as well as the symptoms of tremors, sweats, palpitations, dizziness, shortness of breath, and numbness and tingling in the arms and legs. Cognitive distortions such as fear of scrutiny by others or fear that one is trapped without escape are also common.

Most theories for the biological causes of phobic disorders focus on the dysregulation of internal biogenic amines, or what we call "emotional molecules." Genetic factors also appear to play a role in both specific phobia and social phobia, especially in blood-injection-injury type, where 60 to 75 percent of patients have at least one first-degree relative with the same phobia. Animal and plant type (such as fear of spiders) also seem to have a strong genetic predisposition.

Psychological theories for why we experience phobias range from displacement of intrapsychic conflict (an unresolved psychological stress or trauma manifesting itself as a phobia) to conditioning (learned) paradigms, depending on the therapist's educational background and basic assumptions. Although often widely different, many of these theories capture enough truth of the disorder to guide the clinician to make appropriate treatment decisions. For instance, a behaviorist would classify *phobia* as an unwanted conditioned response to an originally neutral stimulus. Using social phobia as an example, social situations are avoided because of an anxiety response that is experienced in that setting. Previously, the social situation may have never been linked with a feeling of apprehension. The avoidance response is now linked to social situations where it is perceived another attack may occur, and anticipatory anxiety may precede a social engagement by many weeks.

Treatment from this perspective would then focus on de-linking the specific response of anxiety and avoidance from the stimulus (social interaction). A psychoanalyst, on the other hand, would view social anxiety as a symptom of a deeper conflict; for instance, low self-esteem. Treatment would then focus on improving the patient's view of himself.

Many different theories and methods are valid and helpful ways of approaching the treatment of phobias. Here's a brief overview of phobic conditions, followed by a more in-depth treatment of each category:

Agoraphobia: Irrational fear of being in a place where there is no escape (stuck in traffic; boxed in by others at a baseball game; jammed into a crowded bus; stopped in a tunnel or bridge; locked into an airplane). The patient fears having an anxiety attack in this situation that will result in humiliation, incapacitation, or some other catastrophe. Rather than a specific object or situation, agoraphobics fear having the internal symptoms of an anxiety attack and the perceived catastrophic consequences. Because of this, they stay home, making elaborate excuses for why they can't go out and do things. Some become physically ill if they try to leave their home, developing sudden onset of nausea, vomiting, dizziness, and overwhelming dread.

Specific Phobias: Persistent fear of objects or situations, exposure to which causes an immediate anxiety reaction. Situational type phobias, or phobias associated with activities or experiences, commonly include fear of going through a tunnel, taking an elevator, flying, crossing a bridge, vomiting, and having sex. Animal and plant types include fear of germs or certain animals and insects, with onset usually in early childhood. Phobias associated with conditions, emotions, or sensations include fear of heights, pain, fainting, confined or open spaces, failure, laughter, and anger. Natural or environmental type includes fear of storms, heights, water, wind, infinity, fire, and night, and also has its onset in childhood. Blood-injection-injury type frequently involves fear of needles or procedures, while phobias associated with body parts, functions, and afflictions covers a wide range of hypochondriacal and physical fears. Just about any object, color, or substance can be the object of a fear response, such as garlic, dust, anything purple (like Barney), meat, chemicals, pesticides, cars, cemeteries, puppets, meteors, and so on. Lastly, we can develop phobias for people or professions, such as teenagers, women, men, priests, bald people, beggars, dentists (probably really from a blood-injection-injury type fear), and so forth.

In specific phobia, fears are externalized to the object, such as *What if the plane crashes? What if the bee stings me and causes an allergic reaction? What if the escalator stops suddenly and several people tumble on top of me?* This is different from agoraphobia, where the patient fears internal sensations that may lead to the feared "catastrophe," such as *What if I get anxious on the plane and throw up and am humiliated and embarrassed for the rest of the flight?* People with specific phobias can fear internal sensations as well, but their concern is not as overwhelming and is restricted to a single and specific type of situation.

Social Phobia: Specific fear of social or performance situations, especially if loss of face, embarrassment, or causing worry to others is a distinct possibility. The social phobic will avoid situations where they have to meet new people due to an unrealistic fear that they are being scrutinized. For example, a new teacher may dread the first day of school where he will be "looked over" and judged by his new students. This fear of social or performance situations persists despite the awareness of the individual that the fear is excessive and unreasonable. Making presentations, taking oral exams, and attending social events are all painful experiences for the social phobic. One study showed that the No. 1 fear of those surveyed was public speaking, while the number two fear was death. An estimated 10 million Americans suffer from social phobia. It is the most common anxiety disorder and third most common psychiatric disorder behind alcohol/substance abuse and depression. They have fewer social skills than panic patients (who learn to cling to others), and therefore become isolated and depressed more easily. Social phobia usually starts in the teenage years, sometimes after a stressful or humiliating experience. Onset after age 25 is uncommon.

In addition to these three common forms of phobia, a hybrid fourth category should also be mentioned:

Phobias Arising From Underlying Anxiety Disorders: After a careful history, a person's phobia may be determined to arise from an underlying anxiety disorder rather than being a true specific or social phobia.

Paul is a single 37-year-old computer programmer. He had been told by a psychologist that he has obsessive-compulsive disorder (OCD), and came to his physician for medical treatment. He had tried a cognitive behavioral therapy program, but found it was "too much work." Paul obsessed about germs and contamination. He worried that he would get these germs if he touched someone else, even incidentally. He was afraid of just about any object that might carry germs. Anything he might come in contact with needed to be cleaned and re-cleaned. If someone used his bathroom, he made sure it was thoroughly decontaminated before he could use it again. His life was greatly inconvenienced by the need to wash and clean. He estimated that his hands got washed at least 40 times a day.

Predictably, Paul's relationships had not gone well. Within a short period of time, his dates realized he had some real issues about physical contact. And his need to have the surrounding environment sterilized was judged by his friends as just plain weird. Because of a string of rejections, Paul stopped dating, ceased inviting friends over, and quit going to public places ("Because they're dirty," he explained). He became more and more isolated, anxious, and depressed. To soothe his anxious feelings, he turned to alcohol, drinking two bottles of wine at night after work to calm down. His sleep patterns were disrupted by panic attacks early in the morning, and he still felt tired when the alarm went off at 6 a.m.

In addition, Paul admitted to feeling low motivation, and had no passion or interest in things he used to enjoy, such as mountain biking and playing guitar. He had an overwhelming sense of worthlessness and despair, with no feelings of hope for a better life. His work as a programmer was suffering due to increasing problems focusing on this technical and detailed work. He had received a negative report from his supervisor about a recent drop-off in productivity.

Paul's fear of germs might be superficially labeled as a specific phobia of the animal and plant type. But the compulsive behavior of cleaning and washing, as well as the significant dysfunction caused by his anxiety, clearly indicates that his phobia is the manifestation of an underlying anxiety disorder, OCD. In addition, he has developed a substance abuse problem with alcohol, as well as a depressed mood disorder with features of fatigue, low motivation, and severely reduced interest in pleasurable activities. He has acquired a sleep disorder, probably because of anxiety and the disruptive effects alcohol has on sleep patterns. He has found that as the alcohol wears off, he wakes up to face all the anxious feelings he had tried to suppress.

To label Paul's problem as a simple phobia and send him off to therapy would be to miss the primary diagnosis of OCD and ignore the secondary conditions that follow. (In Chapter 7 we will explore the medical plan that got Paul back on track using the symptom-based approach. Happily, after about six weeks of treatment he was nearly free of his fear of germs and had greatly improved his functionality at work and in his social life.)

THE CLOSING WALLS OF AGORAPHOBIA

The latest edition of the *Diagnostic and Statistical Manual of Mental Disorders, DSM-IV* (American Psychiatric Association, 2000) defines agoraphobia as anxiety about being in places or situations from which escape may be difficult because of physical or social constraints (embarrassment) or where help may not be available in the event of a panic attack or panic-like symptoms such as heart palpitations, dizziness, nausea, vomiting, diarrhea, or loss of bladder control. These fears cause the agoraphobic patient to avoid the feared situation or enter it with great discomfort.

Agoraphobia can be divided into two types. One involves a fear of panic attacks, and is called panic disorder with agoraphobia (PDA). To qualify for this diagnosis, one must have random panic attacks that follow no predictable pattern. These panic attacks are characterized as sudden surges of intense fear accompanied by at least four of the following symptoms: palpitations/pounding heart, sensations of shortness of breath or smothering, light-headedness/dizziness/faint feelings, sweating, hot or cold flashes, trembling/shaking, numbness/tingling, choking sensations, nausea/abdominal distress, chest pain/discomfort, feelings of unreality, fear of dying, and fear of going crazy or losing control. People with other phobias fear having a panic attack if confronted with (or while anticipating) the feared object or situation. Agoraphobics with PDA fear having an *unexpected* panic attack.

The next type is agoraphobia without history of panic disorder (AWHPD). This category includes fear of any symptom attack other than panic. Someone with a phobia due to a fear of fainting or a fear of vomiting with no history of panic attacks would be classified in this category.

A succinct definition of agoraphobia is that of Drs. Pollard and Zuercher-White in *The Agoraphobia Workbook* (New Harbinger Publications, 2003):

"Agoraphobia is a maladaptive fear of and desire to avoid situations in which the individual believes a symptom attack may occur and result in incapacitation, humiliation, or some other catastrophe."

Agoraphobia leads to phobic avoidance, which may be limited to a specific situation, or expanded to include any situation that the individual believes could trigger a panic or anxiety attack. In this way, the agoraphobic's options in life become increasingly limited, leading to social isolation and career difficulties.

Agoraphobia is estimated to affect between 2.8 to 5.7 percent of the population (Barlow, 1988). A large percentage of these patients never seek professional help or medical treatment. About three-fourths of agoraphobic patients experience panic attacks, and 60 percent of patients with panic disorder develop agoraphobia. About 65–75 percent of agoraphobic patients are women, presumably because they tend to use avoidance to cope with anxiety, while men more often turn to alcohol and drugs.

Agoraphobia usually develops gradually, starting with a panic or anxiety attack with any number of unpleasant symptoms. From then on, fear of another attack leads to avoidance of a variety of situations that the individual feels might trigger another attack. Repeated, unexpected panic attacks lead to cognitive distortions and conditioned avoidance responses. In addition, abnormalities in norepinephrine, serotonin, and gamma-aminobutyric acid (GABA) neurotransmission may be present. There may be a low level of persistent anticipatory anxiety, where many different situations are entertained as potential threats. The nervous system becomes hyperalert and hypervigilant, focusing intently on every internal symptom and sensation to determine whether it is announcing the onset of another anxiety attack.

The individual may also fear a particular symptom more than the anxiety itself. For instance, the specific symptom of diarrhea, fainting, headache, vomiting, and loss of bladder control are often the focus of the fear response. In these cases, just thinking about the feared symptom may lead to an anxiety attack. Whether the agoraphobic patient fears a specific symptom of a general anxiety attack, it is usually because they perceive a catastrophe will happen as a result of the attack. This anticipated catastrophe might be imagined as public humiliation or shame, a full-blown psychological "breakdown," or a physical event such as heart attack or stroke. Another category is the "spiritual catastrophe," where the person feels they may be judged, punished, or alienated from God or experience some other negative consequence related to religious beliefs or spirituality.

In understanding agoraphobia, it is helpful to begin by identifying the feared symptoms of an anxiety attack as well as the details of the feared catastrophe. It will also be necessary to acknowledge avoidant coping strategies or how the person feels an attack can be prevented by resorting to certain behaviors. Unfortunately, these behaviors and strategies that avoid fear only allow misinterpretations and misperceptions to continue and be reinforced so that the agoraphobia just gets worse over time. Avoidant coping is a useful skill if a real danger exists. But if one's perception of danger is flawed, as in cases of agoraphobia, then avoidance prevents unlearning misperceptions and learning the truth of one's situation. "Primary avoidance" strategies include ways in which the person will avoid completely or endure with great discomfort a particular place or situation. When avoidance is not practical, "secondary avoidance" develops, or so-called "safety behaviors." These can include visiting a feared place only in the company of a trusted friend, entering a feared situation only at particular times of day ("I'm okay in the evening"), and enduring a stressful circumstance only when medicated ("I can get through if I've taken my Xanax").

Understanding our own personal catastrophic thinking, phobic avoidance, and safety behaviors is the key focus of cognitive behavioral therapy designed to overcome this condition. Exposure therapy or "desensitization" can then be utilized, resulting in the emotional learning response that gives deep, long-term resolution of agoraphobic fears. Agoraphobia with panic attacks most often responds to treatment with a selective serotonin reuptake inhibitor (SSRI). Tricyclic antidepressants (TCAs) and monoamine oxidase inhibitors (MAOIs) have also demonstrated efficacy in controlled trials. Benzodiazepines, which stimulate the GABA system, are also beneficial, although their use is limited due to the potential for abuse, especially if a previous history of substance abuse exists. Cognitive behavioral therapy, family therapy, and group therapy are also effective forms of treatment for panic disorder and agoraphobia. Because in real life a complex presentation of symptoms and diagnoses is common, the symptom-based approach to treatment is especially useful (as explained in the next chapter).

An Example of Agoraphobia

Janice is a 35-year-old single mother with a 5-year-old daughter. She suffers from migraine headaches that can be triggered by a number of factors, including hormone changes, lack of sleep, stress, skipping a meal, and even from exposure to fluorescent lights. One time in the supermarket, she found the overhead lights annoying and felt the familiar headache starting. As usual with her migraines, she knew that nausea and even vomiting were secondary symptoms and could occur without much warning. Fearing she might throw up, but having finished her shopping, she had the choice of leaving her cart and going home, or braving the long line at the checker's station and getting her purchases. While standing there in indecision, she began focusing on a particularly disturbing thought: what if she threw up all over the cart or onto the person in front of her? The more she thought of this possibility, the more light-headed and sweaty she felt, until a wave of nausea finally overcame her. The projectile vomit sprayed the checkout counter and the left arm of the bag boy. Horrified, she began crying and shaking. The staff cleaned things up and helped her to a private office where she could recover.

From then on, Janice had a phobia about vomiting in public, especially in the grocery store. But she also worried about having a vomiting attack in the bank, the gas station, the post office, at work, and many other places. She wanted to avoid going out of the house altogether, but she needed to make a living and take care of her daughter. She didn't go back to the market at all, hiring a neighbor to go shopping for her and deliver the groceries to the house twice a week. She endured work and other public places with great discomfort.

Certain behaviors helped her feel safer. She would always ask the location of all the exits and nearest bathrooms—in case of an attack, she wanted to have an "escape plan." She carried crackers and soda in her purse because these had sometimes helped her nausea. She would never eat on the morning she had to go to an unfamiliar building and carried a Walkman so she could distract herself with loud music whenever thoughts of vomiting became obsessive.

For Janice to benefit from therapy, she will first need to identify her fear. There are four components of agoraphobic fear. The first is *the fear of external danger signals.* These are feared situations, places, and activities that signal danger and the possibility of a feared sensation or symptom attack. The second component is *the fear of internal danger signals.* These are feelings and sensations such as heart palpitations, dizziness, difficulty breathing, trembling, and nausea. These sensations trigger the third component, which is *the fear of having a symptom attack.* The sensations just listed will only provoke anxiety if they are seen as precursors to an impending symptom attack. For instance, shortness of breath may be a feared sensation because it may lead to fainting, which is the feared symptom attack. The fourth component of agoraphobic fear is *the feared catastrophe.* This is the final outcome of a symptom attack, and can include such things as embarrassment, humiliation, insanity, heart attack, stroke, or death. What catastrophe does Janice believe will happen? She fears the catastrophe of complete humiliation in front of her neighbors. What about her feared symptom attack? She fears the symptom of vomiting. What internal sensation heralds the possibility of a vomiting attack? The migraine headache. And which external danger signals can we identify in Janice's case? They would include the grocery store, bank, post office, and just about any public building.

Now look at the behaviors that she has adopted to avoid the feared catastrophe. Her *primary avoidance behavior* is complete refusal to show her face in the grocery store where the vomiting occurred. *Secondary avoidance,* or "safety behaviors," include having an escape plan and not eating in advance of a feared situation, as well as keeping soda, crackers, and a Walkman in her purse. These primary and secondary avoidance behaviors will prevent Janice from making any progress in overcoming her case of agoraphobia because they allow and reinforce a false belief that her life will be ruined if she vomits in public. These factors are present in specific and social phobia as well. Being able to specify them for one's own situation is an important step in overcoming the kind of physical and emotional prison Janice experienced.

THE SELECTIVITY OF SPECIFIC PHOBIA

Specific phobia has a female-to-male ratio of 2:1. The age of onset depends on the phobia. For example, animal phobia appears at a mean age of 7 years. Blood-injection-injury phobia starts at a mean age of 9 years, whereas dental phobia appears at a mean age of 10 years and claustrophobia at a mean age of 20 years. Specific phobia can be acquired by conditioning, modeling, traumatic experience, or through a genetic component. Specific phobias usually respond to behavioral therapy. Gradual desensitization, or "exposure therapy," is the most commonly used form of treatment for this disorder. Other treatments include cognitive approaches, relaxation strategies, and breathing control techniques. No controlled studies to date demonstrate the efficacy of psychopharmological intervention, although we certainly have anecdotal experience that points to the usefulness of treating other emotional disorders contributing to the overall phobic vulnerability.

To appreciate the broad range of situations or objects that can be the stimulus of a phobic response, we have grouped the phobias into seven categories. Unavoidably, some overlap between these categories exists, but the groupings are still helpful for organization and purposes of discussion. As you peruse this long list, take note of the fact that many human beings over time have developed specific phobias to just about everything under the sun. You can use this list to check the formal names of phobias which you may be experiencing.

1. Phobias Associated With Activities or Experiences (Situational Type)

As an example of this phobia class, James at 42 years old felt simultaneously confused and embarrassed by his agyrophobia, a fear of crossing streets. As a teenager, he had narrowly avoided death after looking the wrong way before stepping into a London street, where of course the traffic was coming from the opposite direction to what he expected, being a tourist from the United States. James has developed elaborate avoidance strategies, including taking a cab to travel even a block or two and planning his walks with elaborate care to avoid crossing major thoroughfares.

When he stands at the street curb, James feels panic symptoms overwhelm him. These can be lessened only by stepping back from the curb. Only when there is no other alternative does James steel himself to cross a street, but only after taking several minutes to look up and down the street for any sign of traffic. He typically waits until cars are a block or more away before scampering as quickly as he can across the street, all the while suffering phobic symptoms of anxiety and panic.

Phobias associated with activities and experiences include:

Ablutophobia (bathing)

Achluophobia (darkness)

Agyrophobia (crossing streets)

Amaxophobia (being in or riding in vehicles)

Ambulophobia (walking)

Aviatophobia (flying)

Cathisophobia (sitting)

Chorophobia (dancing)

Cibophobia (food or eating)

Climacophobia (falling down stairs)

Clinophobia (going to bed)

Coitophobia (sexual intercourse)

Deipnophobia (dining and dinner conversation)

Dipsophobia (drinking)

Emetophobia (vomiting)

Ergophobia (work)

Gametophobia (marriage)

Genophobia (sex)

Gephyrophobia (crossing bridges)

Gerascophobia (growing old)

Glossophobia (speaking in public)

Hamartophobia (sinning)

Harpaxophobia (being robbed)

Hodophobia (road travel)

Hypnophobia (sleep)

Maieusiophobia (childbirth)

Malaxophobia (foreplay or other play associated with sex)

Merinthophobia (being bound)

Neophobia (anything new)

Obesophobia (gaining weight)

Ombrophobia (being rained on)

Onomatophobia (hearing a certain word or name)

Panphobia (everything)

Panthophobia (suffering and disease)

Peccatophobia (sinning or imaginary crimes)

Peniaphobia (poverty)

Phagophobia (swallowing, eating, or being eaten)

Phalacrophobia (becoming bald)

Philemaphobia or philematophobia (kissing)

Philophobia (falling in love or being in love)

Phobophobia (phobias)

Plutophobia (wealth)

Pluviophobia (rain or of being rained on)

Pneumatiphobia (spirits)

Pnigophobia or pnigerophobia (choking or being smothered)

Pocrescophobia (gaining weight)

Poinephobia (punishment)

Psellismophobia (stuttering)

Pteromerhanophobia (flying)

Rhypophobia (defecation)

Rhytiphobia (getting wrinkles)

Sarmassophobia (foreplay or other play associated with sex)

Sciophobia or sciaphobia (shadows)

Scolionophobia (school)

Scopophobia or Scoptophobia (being seen or stared at)

Scotophobia (darkness)

Selaphobia (light flashes)

Siderodromophobia (trains, railroads, or train travel)

Sitophobia or sitiophobia (food or eating)

Somniphobia (sleep)

Soteriophobia (dependence on others)

Tachophobia (speed)

Taphephobia or taphophobia (being buried alive or of cemeteries)

Testophobia (taking tests)

Thanatophobia or thantophobia (death or dying)

Tocophobia (pregnancy or childbirth)

Urophobia (urine or urinating)

Virginitiphobia (rape)

Zelophobia (jealousy)

2. Phobias Associated With Animals and Plants

As an example of this phobia class, consider Cindy's case. She developed ornithophobia (a fear of birds) in young adulthood after seeing Alfred Hitchcock's *The Birds*. At first she avoided parks and public buildings known to have flocks of birds, especially crows and pigeons. But soon she found that walking on a sidewalk was a high-risk activity. Even a single bird fluttering out of a tree and landing in front of her would elicit a strong startle and scream response. Others would stop what they were doing to try to figure out what had frightened her. Of course, they could not see anything that could have been perceived as a threat. This would lead to mild embarrassment, and she would quickly walk away with her head down.

If she had been more vulnerable to fearing the internal sensations of her heart racing or the scrutiny of others, Cindy might easily have developed agoraphobia over time. But she didn't care all that much what other's thought, knowing they would soon turn their attention to something else. And she knew her heart would not be damaged by the experience. Her specific phobia of birds did, however, cause her to turn down certain activities and opportunities. She would turn down any invitation to eat outdoors, where seagulls or pigeons might fly in or be underfoot. She did not go to outdoor concerts, visit parks, and even refused to travel to Italy because she had previously seen flocks of birds around the churches and cathedrals on a TV travel program.

Phobias associated with animals and plants include:

Acarophobia (itching caused by insects)

Agrizoophobia (wild animals)

Ailurophobia (cats)

Alektorophobia (chickens)

Apiphobia (bees)

Arachnophobia (spiders)

Batrachophobia (amphibians, including frogs, newts, and salamanders)

Blennophobia (slime)

Botanophobia (plants)

Bufonophobia (toads)

Cnidophobia (insect stings)

Cynophobia (dogs or rabies)

Dendrophobia (trees)

Doraphobia (fur or animal skins)

Elurophobia (cats)

Entomorphobia (insects)

Equinophobia (horses)

Galeophobia (cats)

Helminthophobia (being infested with worms)

Herpetophobia (reptiles or creepy-crawly things)

Hippophobia (horses)

Hylophobia (forests)

Icthyophobia (fish)

Insectophobia (insects)

Isopterophobia (termites)

Lachanophobia (vegetables)

Microbiophobia (microbes)

Misophobia (contamination by germs or dirt)

Mottephobia (moths)

Musophobia or muriphobia (mice)

Myrmecophobia (ants)

Ornithophobia (birds)

Ophidiophobia (snakes)

Ostraconophobia (shellfish)

Parasitophobia (parasites)

Pediculophobia (lice)

Scoleciphobia (worms)

Selachophobia (sharks)

Sheksophobia (wasps)

Spermatophobia (germs)

Suriphobia (mice)

Taeniophobia (tapeworms)

Taurophobia (bulls)

3. Phobias Associated With Conditions, Emotions, or Sensations

As an example of this phobia class, consider chiraptophobia, the fear of being touched. A person with this phobia may only fear being touched in a certain area of their body. Erica was a patient being seen for her routine physical. When the physician reached from behind with no warning to feel her thyroid gland, her reflex reaction was a sharp elbow to the examiner's stomach. As he caught his breath, Erica apologized and explained that she had a severe phobia about being touched around her neck. She had no idea why, but remembered this fear existed from early childhood. A few weeks later Erica's mother, also a patient, was visiting for a routine check. She spoke freely about Erica's fear. Her best guess was that Erica's older brother had repeatedly choked her as a child when they were left alone. She had heard Erica's screaming and crying when he finally let go. Erica had experienced complete loss of control, not being able to stop the attack or know when it would finally end. Even in adulthood, her "elbow-jerk" reaction attested to the deep emotional trauma that these experiences had inflicted.

Phobias associated with conditions, emotions, or sensations include:

Acrophobia (heights)

Agateophobia (insanity)

Agliophobia (pain)

Amnesiphobia (amnesia)

Amychophobia (being scratched)

Anemophobia (feeling air drafts)

Anginophobia (angina, physical pressure, or choking)

Angrophobia (anger or becoming angry)

Anuptaphobia (staying single)

Aphenphosmphobia (being touched)

Astenophobia (fainting or weakness)

Ataxiophobia (muscular incoordination)

Ataxophobia (disorder or untidiness)

Atelophobia (imperfection)

Athazagoraphobia (being forgotten or forgetting)

Atychiphobia (failure)

Autodysomophobia (one's own odor, real or imagined)

Batophobia (heights or being close to tall buildings)

Bromidrosiphobia (body smells)

Cacophobia (ugliness)

Catagelophobia (being ridiculed)

Cherophobia (gaiety)

Chiraptophobia (being touched)

Claustrophobia (confined spaces)

Cleithrophobia (being locked in an enclosed space)

Dementophobia (insanity)

Dinophobia (dizziness or whirlpools)

Diplophobia (double vision)

Enosioophobia (having committed an unpardonable sin)

Frigophobia (cold or cold things)

Geliophobia (laughter)

Haphephobia (being touched)

Hedonophobia (feeling pleasure)

Hormephobia (shock)

Homophobia (homosexuality)

Illyngophobia (vertigo)

Kainolophobia (anything new)

Kenophobia (voids or empty spaces)

Kinetophobia (movement or motion)

Kopophobia (fatigue)

Ligyrophobia (loud noises)

Merinthophobia (being bound or tied up)

Monophobia (solitude or being alone)

Obesophobia (gaining weight or being fat)

Olfactophobia or osmophobia (smells)

Ophthalmophobia (being stared at)

Photophobia (light)

Phonophobia (noises or voices)

Pnigophobia (choking or being smothered)

Scotophobia (darkness)

Somniphobia (sleep)

Symmetrophobia (symmetry)

Thanatophobia (death or dying)

Thermophobia (heat)

Xerophobia (dryness)

Zelophobia (jealousy)

4. Phobias Associated With Objects, Colors, and Substances

As an example of this phobia class is John's case. John was a sharp university student getting his Ph.D. in environmental sciences at Stanford. During the course of his studies, he developed chemophobia, a fear of chemicals. Seeing the effects of toxic chemical waste dumps on the health of community residents had a deep impact on him. He began eating organic foods that had not been treated with any pesticides, which meant he felt uncomfortable eating out in restaurants where he was not sure how thoroughly they had washed the produce. He stopped driving a car and rode his bike instead, fearing the chemicals in the petroleum products were making him ill. In fact, if he perceived he had been exposed to some chemical agent, John would suddenly feel physical symptoms of chemical toxicity. He knew the symptoms well from his classes: nausea, headaches, stomach pain, muscle pain, and so on. Even if it turned out he hadn't been exposed, he got the symptoms anyway.

When he found out that the State of California was going to spray wide areas with pesticide to eradicate the fruit fly, John had to stop school to spend a few months with his sister on the east coast. Even this highly intelligent, rational scientist could not overcome his irrational fears, letting this phobia control his life.

Phobias associated with objects, colors, and substances include:

Aichmophobia (needles)

Alliumphobia (garlic)

Amathophobia (dust)

Atephobia (ruins)

Aulophobia (flutes)

Aurophobia (gold)

Bathmophobia (stairs)

Carnophobia (meat)

Catoptrophobia (mirrors)

Chemophobia (chemicals)

Chirophobia (hands)

Chronomentrophobia (clocks)

Cometophobia (comets)

Coimetrophobia (cemeteries)

Crystallophobia (glass or crystals)

Cyberphobia (computers)

Cyclophobia (bicycles)

Enetrophobia (pins)

Hoplophobia (firearms)

Hydrargyophobia (mercurial
medicines)

Iophobia (poison)

Metallophobia (metal)

Meteorophobia (meteors)

Methyphobia (alcohol)

Motorphobia (cars)

Nephophobia (clouds)

Ochophobia (vehicles)

Odonotophobia (teeth)

Oenophobia (wines)

Papryophobia (paper)

Pediophobia (dolls)

Placophobia (tombstones)

Pogonophobia (beards)

Porphyrophobia (the color purple)

Parmacophobia (drugs)

Proctophobia (rectums)

Pupaphobia (puppets)

Rupophobia (dirt)

Scatophobia (fecal matter)

Selenophobia (the moon)

Siderophobia (stars)

Telephonophobia (telephones)

Theatrophobia (theaters)

Vestiphobia (clothing)

Xanthophobia (the color yellow)

Xylophobia (wooden objects)

Xyrophobia (razors)

5. Phobias Associated With Natural or Environmental Phenomena

As an example of this phobia class, take Trent's case. Trent carried with him a burdensome fear of atomic explosions (atomosophobia) engendered during his elementary school years in the 1950s, when he was forced to view horrific films of Hiroshima and Nagasaki, along with "public awareness" films showing mushroom clouds and guided missiles. Traumatized by these images as a child, Trent now reacts with sudden and overwhelming panic to the appearance of a thunderhead cloud on the horizon or a loud, unexplained boom of any kind. In the presence of such stimuli, his thoughts turn obsessively to the possibility of nuclear attack and the imminent arrival of a shock wave or firestorm. He typically rushes to the nearest radio or TV to reassure himself that no such attack has taken place.

Phobias associated with natural or environmental phenomena include:

Ancraphobia (wind)

Antlophobia (floods)

Aperiophobia (infinity)

Astraphobia (thunder and
lightning)

Atomosophobia (atomic explosions)

Barophobia (gravity)

Brontophobia (thunder and lightning)

Chronophobia (time)

Cryophobia (extreme ice, frost, or cold)

Eosophobia (dawn or daylight)

Hygrophobia (dampness or moisture)

Kosmikophobia (cosmic phenomena)

Lilapsophobia (tornadoes or hurricanes)

Noctiphobia (night)

Ombrophobia (rain or being rained on)

Potophobia (running water)

Pyrophobia (fire)

Sciophobia (shadows)

Spacephobia (outer space)

Thalassophobia (sea)

Uranophobia (heaven)

6. Phobias Associated With People or Professions

An example of this phobia type is the case of Andrew. Andrew fears bald people (peladophobia). As a child, he inadvertently insulted a bald man in a grocery store and was promptly clapped on the ears by the old man and screamed at. Andrew now turns away from any bald person he sees approaching on the street. He does whatever he can to avoid dealing with bald people in his workplace, even going as far as turning down a promotion because it meant working for a bald boss. When he must face a bald person he feels growing waves of panic and often must make up lame excuses to get out of the presence of that person, if only long enough to calm his symptoms and go back into the encounter to finish it as quickly as possible.

Andrew's most recent phobic dilemma has to do with his own receding hairline. As he looks in the mirror each morning, he sees more and more of the dreaded signs of baldness that he has learned to abhor in others.

Phobias associated with people or professions include:

Androphobia (men)

Anthrophobia (society)

Apotemnophobia (people with amputations)

Bogyphobia (bogeyman)

Caligynephobia (beautiful women)

Coulrophobia (clowns)

Demonophobia (demons)

Denophobia (dentists)

Enochlophobia (crowds)

Ephebiphobia (teenagers)

Gynephobia (women)

Hagiophobia (saints)

Hierophobia (priests)

Hobophobia (beggars or bums)

Novercaphobia (stepmothers)

Parthenophobia (young girls)

Pedophobia (children)

Peladophobia (bald people)

Pentheraphobia (mothers-in-law)

Politicophobia (politicians)

Soceraphobia (parents-in-law)

Tyrannophobia (tyrants)

Xenophobia (strangers or
  foreigners)

7. Phobias Associated With Body Parts, Functions, and Afflictions (Blood-Injection-Injury Type)

As an example of this phobia class, consider the case of Rachel. Rachel hates hypodermic needles used for injections and blood work (trypanophobia) to the point that she despairs of ever getting married because a blood test is required in her state. She specifically worries not so much about the prick of pain involved in a skin puncture by a needle, but about the imagined catastrophe of a needle tip breaking off inside her body and then traveling somehow to her heart and killing her. Over the years she has changed physicians several times. She typically leaves her doctor when a blood workup, flu injection, or other shot is ordered. She is too embarrassed to explain her fears to her doctor, so she simply does not show up for the injection and starts afresh with a new doctor. At this point Rachel has developed a gallbladder condition that will require relatively minor arthroscopic surgery—involving, of course, the use of a needle to introduce anesthesia. Rachel has endured several painful gallbladder attacks rather than proceeding with the operation, which will bring her comfort and potentially save her life if her gallbladder condition worsens.

Phobias associated with body parts, functions, and afflictions (blood-injection-injury type) include:

Aeronausiphobia (vomiting
  secondary to airsickness)

Albuminurophobia (kidney
  disease)

Ankylophobia (joint immobility)

Cardiophobia (heart)

Coitophobia (sexual intercourse)

Coprastasophobia (constipation)

Coprophobia (feces)

Defecaloesiophobia (painful bowel
  movements)

Dipsophobia (drinking)

Emetophobia (vomiting)

Epistaxiophobia (nosebleeds)

Eruotophobia (female genitalia)

Genophobia (sex)

Gerontophobia (old people or
  growing old)

Gymnophobia (nudity)

Hemophobia (blood)

Hypnophobia (sleep or being hypnotized)

Ithyphallophobia (male genitalia)

Lockiophobia (childbirth)

Nosophobia (becoming ill)

Ommetaphobia (eyes)

Oneirophobia (dreams)

Rhypophobia (defecation)

Sitophobia (eating)

Tomophobia (surgical operations)

Trichopathophobia (hair)

Trypanophobia (injections)

Urophobia (urinating)

Vaccinophobia (vaccination)

FEARS ASSOCIATED WITH SOCIAL PHOBIA

There are two distinct types of social anxiety disorder (SAD)—generalized and nongeneralized. Generalized is the most severe form and is associated with greater impairment because the anxiety is pervasive and occurs in most if not all social and performance situations. The nongeneralized subtype is limited to public speaking or other performance situations. Although usually less disabling, it can still lead to significant underachievement at work or school. Most social phobias begin before age 20. Patients may describe difficulties with speaking in public, eating or drinking in a public place, participating in group meetings, using public restrooms, and meeting new people at parties or social events. Social phobics may also fear confrontation, interaction with authority figures, and being the center of attention, as when the teacher calls on them to stand up and answer a question. Fear of scrutiny by others or of being embarrassed or humiliated is described most often by people with social phobia. The initial cause of social phobia may be a traumatic social experience. Other times, the individual lacks the social skills that allow successful social interaction. A series of negative experiences and rejection over time may lead to social phobia in this case.

These individuals often possess a hypersensitivity to rejection, perhaps related to dysfunction in their serotonin or dopamine neurochemical systems. Current thought points to an interaction between biological, genetic, and personality factors and environmental events. Both medical treatment and psychotherapy are useful in treating social phobia. The most widely used medications used and approved for social phobias are the SSRIs. Failing this, the patient may respond to a high-potency benzodiazepine. Beta-blockers have been used successfully for the treatment of performance anxiety on an as-needed basis. Short-acting benzodiazepines have a high potential for abuse, as does alcohol, in this patient group. Medication can often be tapered gradually and discontinued in patients receiving appropriate therapy.

Distribution of Social Phobia in the Population

Social anxiety disorder (SAD) is the most common anxiety disorder and the third most common mental health disorder, behind major depression and alcohol dependence. The lifetime chance of getting SAD is between 7 to 13 percent. The mean age of onset is 15.5 years (Schneier et al. 1992). Many patients report being shy as young children, and then becoming aware of their anxiety when starting formal schooling. Biologically based temperamental factors during childhood, such as behavioral inhibition (to be discussed shortly), may predispose some children to the development of SAD. The course of SAD is generally long, lasting an average of 25 years, with low rates of recovery (DeWit et al. 1999).

The observation that SAD symptoms seem to improve in older adults may me attributable to the fact that these adults may be able to afford the luxury of insulating themselves from the phobic stimuli. They are no longer the subject of scrutiny in school or the workplace. Younger adults may find a lifestyle that allows their avoidance to go unnoticed by marrying a social phobic, staying single, or choosing a job that requires little social interaction. Although women are more likely to get the disorder, men are more likely to seek treatment. This discrepancy may be due to social expectations of society and the workplace and gender roles, with symptoms causing more impairment for men than women (Weinstock 1999). The majority of individuals with SAD are single.

The disorder has also been associated with increased difficulties in school, lower educational achievement, lower socioeconomic status, more unstable employment history, and elevated rates of financial dependency. SAD has also been associated with several childhood risk factors, including parental marital conflict, frequent moves, and absence of a close, trusting relationship with an adult. There is a high rate of other co-existing psychiatric illnesses in SAD patients, with 81 percent reporting at least one other lifetime psychiatric diagnosis and 48 percent experiencing 3 other diagnoses. Of SAD patients, 57 percent admitted to having another anxiety disorder, 41 percent a mood disorder, and 40 percent comorbid substance abuse. Individuals with SAD frequently use alcohol to self-medicate in order to decrease anticipatory anxiety and reduce avoidance of feared social and/or performance situations. You have no doubt encountered an acquaintance who needed to "down a few brewskies" before a party to feel comfortable mingling with new people. Many famous stage and screen actors have fallen into the trap of needing a stiff drink (or two or three) before the curtain rises. Peter O'Toole immediately comes to mind.

Early Risk Factors for Social Phobia

The fears of socially phobic youth are similar to those of adults. They include fears, in social or performance situations, of being confused, blushing, doing something embarrassing, being judged stupid or weak, or having a panic attack (Essau et al. 1999). The early onset of social anxiety will likely lead to pronounced problems in adulthood. This is because of the disruptive effects of anxiety disorders on the emotionally sensitive and cognitively naïve mind of a child. In addition, by the very nature of their awkward behavior, these children are more likely to have adverse social experiences that amplify their discomfort and fear. Clearly it would be of great benefit to find ways to intervene early with this disorder as soon as it is first suspected.

Early intervention, however, requires an understanding of the precursors and risk factors for this disorder. Among these factors are family genetics, temperament, parenting, information processing, social learning, and peer relationships.

The generalized subtype of SAD appears to have a stronger familial inheritance than discreet, or nongeneralized, social phobia. Not surprisingly, the familial risk for generalized social phobia appears to overlap with avoidant personality disorder (APD). In their family study, Stein and colleagues found that 74 percent of those with generalized social anxiety met the criteria for APD (Stein et al. 1998). Twin studies allow us to parse the relative contributions of genetic and environmental influences and provide estimates of heritability. In studies on 1,000 female twin pairs and 1,200 male twin pairs, Kendler and colleagues (Kendler et al. 1992–1999) were able to estimate a heritability of 50 percent for social phobia. It did not seem to matter if the twins were raised apart or in the same home environment. This finding weighs against the hypothesis that social anxiety is acquired through modeling or social learning within the family. Instead, Kendler and colleagues (Kendler et al. 1999) have suggested that phobias develop when an inherited phobia proneness is activated by exposure to specific environmental stimuli. On the other hand, other studies have suggested a role for shared family environment in the development of social phobia. Lieb and colleagues (2000) found that parental anxiety and parenting style were associated with social phobia in offspring.

The fact that social phobics usually have one or more other psychiatric diagnoses may also be explained by genetics. Kendler and colleagues reported evidence for an inherited "phobia proneness" with shared genetic influences on agoraphobia, social phobia, and specific phobias. This genetic liability to phobic disorders seems to overlap with that of panic disorder and bulimia. Overall, family studies have suggested that social phobia is inherited separately from panic disorder and other phobic disorders, while twin studies suggest overlapping genetic influences.

Behavioral Inhibition and Social Phobia

Shyness and behavioral inhibition (BI) in particular are developmental risk factors for social phobia. The best studied temperamental precursor to the development of social phobia is BI, defined as "behavioral inhibition to the unfamiliar." First described by Jerome Kagan and colleagues at Harvard University, BI represents an enduring tendency to exhibit caution, restraint, and reticence in situations that are novel or unfamiliar. Inhibited toddlers may cling to parents when faced with unfamiliar adults or peers, or refuse to approach new toys or new settings. As the child matures, he or she may show quiet restraint and a hesitancy to smile, approach, or initiate conversations with new peers or adults. Older children with BI may exhibit inhibition in group situations, such as keeping to themselves. Children with extreme BI are likely to remain inhibited over the course of their entire childhood, and most maintain their cautiousness and restraint as adults. Kagan and his colleagues have hypothesized that the BI reflex lowered the threshold to the limbic and sympathetic nervous systems arousal in response to novelty. There appears to be a higher reactivity of the amygdala and its projections to the striatum, hypothalamus, sympathetic chain, and cardiovascular system in individuals with BI.

Others have suggested that BI might be caused by increased activations of right brain centers involved in the "withdrawal response," and a decreased activation of left brain centers involved in the "approach response." Inhibited children have been shown to have increased activation in the right hemisphere of the brain and decreased activation of the left hemisphere (Calkins et al. 1996; Davidson 1994; Schmidt et al. 1999). According to Kagan, children with BI are significantly more likely to develop social phobia. In his studies, the most common fears of children with social phobia were speaking in front of the class, speaking with strangers, being called on in class, and being placed in a crowd of people. The familial nature of social phobia is further demonstrated by a study showing that parents of children identified as being inhibited have a higher rate of social phobia (Rosenbaum et al. 1991). In another study (Cooper and Eke 1999), shy 4-year-olds had mothers with a nearly eight-fold increase in lifetime social phobia compared to children without shyness. It should be noted that the majority of inhibited children did not develop social phobia. Although BI may be a predisposing factor, it by no means ensures that a child with this temperamental marker will develop social phobia.

Parenting and Family Environment Factors

The data on parental influence over the development of social phobia is sparse; however, it appears that parenting styles do influence its course. A parent who encourages their child to take small risks when facing feared situations may be able to reduce the child's anxiety and avoidance. But if the parent avoids the feared situation themselves or reacts with alarm, the child might learn to avoid uncomfortable situations. Because of this observation, cognitive behavioral therapy (CBT) for childhood anxiety disorders often adds a parental component to improve the outcome (Barrett et al. 1996). Anxious parents should undergo anxiety-management training to maximize the benefit of CBT to their children with anxiety. In addition, well-meaning and responsive parents may unwittingly facilitate their child's avoidance of social situations if they respond to the child's clingy behavior by protecting and comforting them, rather than forcing them to face the feared situation despite their discomfort. Many studies have shown that parents who exert maximal control over a child's activities and decisions, especially if devoid of emotional warmth, predispose the child to psychopathology. Such parenting negatively influences the child's sense of being able to control his or her own environment. In addition, parental restrictiveness, punitiveness, and inconsistency seem to contribute to a child's expectation of negative outcomes. Several researchers have come to the conclusion that infants whose parents are appropriately responsive (e.g., warm, engaged) develop secure attachments with good outcomes (e.g., self-confidence, good peer relations) later in childhood, while children whose parents display rejecting, interfering, or ignoring behavior may develop insecure or anxious attachment behaviors (Ainsworth, 1982; Blehar, Lieberman, and Ainsworth, 1977). In another study, patients with social phobia reported that their parents evinced high concern with the opinions of others, shame of their shyness, and shame of a poor performance (Caster, Inderbitzen, and Hope 1999). Children who experience criticism, rejection, or shaming may become preoccupied with evaluative comments, leading to generalized fear of negative evaluation, self-consciousness, and avoidance of social scrutiny (Bruch, 1989).

The Role of Anxious Cognitions in Social Phobia

Anxious cognitions are thoughts, beliefs, and feelings resulting from the interaction of biological, social, and psychological systems. When a person with a phobia fails to accurately assess these cognitions, the anxiety intensifies and is only relieved by an avoidant or defensive response. Not only do anxious thoughts themselves perpetuate the phobia, but the avoidant behaviors that follow prevent the individual from experiences that would disprove their fears, thereby ensuring that the phobia will persist. It has been proposed that shyness, specific social phobia, generalized social phobia, and avoidant personality disorder have similar cognitive antecedents, and belong along a continuum of "concerns about social evaluation" (Rapee and Heimberg 1997). Individuals with these conditions assume that others are inherently critical and likely to view them negatively. At the same time, those with social anxiety attach great importance to being viewed positively by others. It is common for socially phobic individuals to enter a social situation with a mental representation of their external appearance and behavior as an audience might see them. Of course, they assume that this audience is looking to find fault and is prone to negative scrutiny. The social phobic focuses a great deal of attention on the internal representation of their self-image and is constantly looking for threats from the environment, such as signs of disapproval or rejection. To them, people at the party are a threatening audience rather than new friends to get to know and enjoy. It is no wonder that with all the energy expended searching for threatening clues and avoiding uncomfortable interaction, the social phobic's negative expectation of poor social performance are realized and reconfirmed. Cognitive therapy must be directed at correcting anxious perceptions before exposure therapy can disconfirm negative beliefs and expectations.

Conditioning Experiences and Social Phobia

Many people with social phobia recall a defining embarrassing or humiliating experience associated with the onset of their disorder. In one study, 58 percent of social phobics could identify a traumatic social experience near or at the onset of their illness (Ost, 1985). Another study found that 44 percent of patients with social phobia reported a traumatic conditioning experience that started their symptoms (Stemberg et al. 1995). Most often, these experiences occurred during adolescence, a time when individuals are socially awkward and more vulnerable to embarrassment. It is also clear that indirect experiences can lead to conditioned fears. Ost reported that 16 percent of those with social anxiety developed their phobia by observing others undergoing traumatic social experiences, and 3 percent of his sample acquired social phobia after hearing about another's traumatic experience. Clearly there must be an underlying vulnerability to anxiety to begin with, with the direct or indirect traumatic experience serving as the trigger for the development of social phobia. Temperamental factors and cognitive distortions already present may allow the trauma to be magnified and internalized. Because the condition of social phobia may have already been present before the remembered conditioning experience, it is possible that many recalled incidence may represent early manifestations of the disorder rather than causal events.

The Influence of Peers on Social Phobia

Peer relations in childhood appear to have significant impact on the development of social phobia. As a person with anxiety and social awkwardness will likely get negative feedback in the form of peer rejection or neglect, that then exacerbates and maintains the anxiety. Children who are socially anxious generally perceive that their peer acceptance is low and report more negative interaction with peers, such as being teased or having an enemy at school (Ginsburg et al. 1998). Similarly, very shy or withdrawn children were viewed by their peers as less approachable, less socially competent, and less socially desirable (Evans 1993). These children often are the targets of victimization by the schoolyard bullies. Once neglect, rejection, or victimization occurs, they affect the socially anxious child's sense of self-worth. Many children with a history of peer rejection and teasing will blame themselves for having internal character deficiencies. These children experience increased loneliness, higher levels of social anxiety and avoidance, and lower self-esteem. Children who blamed their *behavior* for difficulties with peers rather than their character *did not* experience these problems (Graham and Juvonen 1998). Understanding the role of peer influences in the development of social anxiety may help educators create preventive interventions for at-risk youth.

As a case in point, Margery is a 25-year-old college student with an incapacitating problem of blushing and sweating profusely in specific social situations. The phobic response was triggered by any situation where she became the center of attention. Whether it was a single person calling out her name in the grocery store to say hello or a teacher calling on her to respond to a question in front of the class, Margery would immediately feel the blood rushing to her cheeks while the sweat drenched her blouse. Her horror that others might think negatively of her (thinking that she is weak, insecure, not prepared, stupid) prevented Margery from taking many of the participation-type classes that were necessary for her degree in communications. She found herself falling behind in her academic program.

On her initial evaluation, it turned out that her social phobia had started at age 15 when her parents moved her from an all-girl's high school to an all-boy's school that had recently become coeducational. She was one of five girls admitted that year, and her parents were especially proud because of the high academic standards and reputation of this new school. Margery, however, soon learned to dread going to school, where she found herself the center of all the adolescent boys' attentions. She hunched her shoulders to make her developing breasts less apparent, which she perceived, probably correctly, to be the focus of their scrutiny. The last thing she wanted was to be stared at, so she made all attempts to avoid anything that would draw attention to her. The same fear of scrutiny and attention had followed her full-force into adulthood, and was now threatening her academic progress.

Margery went through several sessions of cognitive behavioral therapy, which helped reduce the anxiety in some situations. However, in performance situations in front of her class, her symptoms remained intolerable. The administration of a low dose SSRI medication (Paxil) caused sedation and made her sex life a problem, she having difficutly reaching orgasm. We therefore tried a low dose beta-blocker (propanolol 10mg) to be taken 30 minutes before the feared social situation. For extra assurance, we also prescribed Drysol, a powerful antiperspirant, to be used on the palms of her hands and under the arms only on the morning of a presentation. Although this approach helped with her difficulties at school, Margery still can't prevent the automatic blushing response when someone unexpectedly calls her name. For this, she will need ongoing exposure therapy to unlearn this emotional response.

DETERRENCE AND PREVENTION OF PHOBIC STIMULI

Because of the power of emotional learning in early childhood, when the emotional mind is not informed by a developed rational mind, overwhelming exposure to a frightening experience may predispose a child to the development of phobic symptoms. Being lunged at by a large, fiercely barking dog may make a big impression that is the seed of an animal phobia, for instance. Parental reactivity may also play a part in acquiring phobias in this age group. Patty, the wife of Dr. Gardner, feels her fear of water started as a very young girl. She remembers how her mother, who also has a fear of water, would forcefully pull her back if she ventured too close to a pond, pool, or water's edge. She remembers seeing the fear in her mother's eyes and trembling of her hands, as if she had just avoided a potentially fatal car accident. This conditioning of the fear response effectively ingrained the water phobia so that Patty refuses to learn to swim.

If recognized early, intervention with psychotherapy in the early stages of symptom development may be beneficial in preventing a worsening of the symptoms and the development of a lifetime phobia.

COMPLICATIONS OF UNTREATED PHOBIAS

If left untreated, phobias can result in tremendous loss of potential and quality of life for the individual. This is especially true of agoraphobia and social phobia. As the ability to work and relate to other people becomes impaired, relationship and financial stressors take their toll. The inevitable isolation commonly leads to substance abuse, especially with alcohol and sedatives. Patients with specific phobias are also impaired, but can usually live around the phobic stimulus without drawing too much attention to their dysfunction. But imagine not being able to go into a building (acrophobia), a small elevator (claustrophobia), or even your backyard (e.g., fear of snakes or insects). Consider also the dilemma of those phobic sufferers whose career has stagnated or collapsed due to a fear of flying, crossing bridges, eating in restaurants, or using public restrooms. Although lost potential is difficult to quantify, it is still part of the high cost of phobias to individuals, their families, and society.

Medical and Legal Pitfalls
Associated With Social Phobia

An estimation of the cost of phobias must include medical and legal problems that can be directly attributed to the condition. Patients with agoraphobia and social phobia have a higher risk of social isolation, substance abuse, and suicidal ideation. Agoraphobic patients may be housebound and unable to seek medical care for serious problems. Also, because anxiety and panic attack symptoms resemble those found in life-threatening medical emergencies such as heart attack and stroke, significant hospital resources must be utilized to rule out these possibilities when a patient presents to the emergency room.

A Prognosis for Those With Phobias

Fortunately, most patients do respond to treatment, with good resolution of symptoms. Patients with specific phobias usually achieve the highest level of functioning, while agoraphobics and social phobics may continue to combat residual symptoms and run a greater risk of relapse, even after successful treatment. A particularly difficult problem is the social phobic with poor social skills. But with proper learning of these skills, even so-called "geeks" and "nerds" can overcome social phobia.

Unfortunately, the vast majority of patients with these disorders never seek professional help. Whether they cannot afford it, have no time for it, feel it would be useless for them, feel ashamed to admit their "weakness," or the have a fear of health professionals, most people suffer silently with these problems their entire lives. Their spouses and children suffer as well, both financially and emotionally.

What is needed is a straightforward, affordable, nonjudgmental, and practical method that can bring the patient into the loop of understanding so that the process of restoring control and functionality can begin. This book aspires to fulfill this purpose.

The following diagram of intersecting spheres shows the differential diagnosis of phobia so that a patient can quickly self-diagnose between agoraphobia, agoraphobia with panic disorder, social phobia, and specific phobia. In addition, common features that are shared among the phobias are made clear.

DIAGNOSTIC CRITERIA OF PHOBIC DISORDERS

SOCIAL PHOBIA

Involves fear of social or performance situations, especially if loss of face or deep embarrassment is possible. Social situations are avoided due to an unrealistic fear of scrutiny. It usually starts in adolescence or childhood after a stressful or humiliating experience. Onset after age 25 is uncommon.

AGORAPHOBIA

The irrational fear of having a symptom attack in a situation where escape may be difficult. The agoraphobic fears that the anxiety attack will lead to humiliation, incapacitation, or some catastrophy, such as a stroke, heart attack, loss of sanity, or even death. It usually starts in adulthood, and some difficult cases may become housebound.

AGORAPHOBIA WITH PANIC DISORDER

In addition, there are unpredictable and recurrent panic attacks.

PHOBIAS: COMMON FEATURES

All phobias are exaggerated fear responses. The symptoms experienced during phobic anxiety are common to all phobias because they are caused by the same sympathetic nervous system activation. These symptoms include irregular or fast heartbeats, chills, sweats, hot flashes, shortness of breath, nausea, abdominal pain, faintness or dizziness, shakiness, choking sensations, chest discomfort, numbness and tingling, thoughts of doom or death, feeling of unreality or being detached from oneself.

PHOBIA DUE TO AN UNDERLYING ANXIETY DISORDER

For example, OCD patients may have a phobia involving contamination; GAD patients are often shy and have features of social phobia; those with Panic Disorder may fear going crazy, but only during a panic attack.

SPECIFIC PHOBIA

Persistant fears of specific objects or situations, exposure to which causes an immediate anxiety response. Those with purely a specific phobia do not go on to develop an agoraphobic fear of having the anxiety response, so the person is only limited when it comes to their specific fear. Often starts in childhood.

Gardner and Bell, 2004

Chapter 6

ANXIETY AND MOOD DISORDERS UNDERLYING PHOBIAS

This chapter answers four questions:

1. What emotional illnesses and conditions often precede and accompany phobias?
2. What factors create a vulnerability to phobias?
3. How does underlying depression in its various forms influence phobic experience?
4. How do anxiety conditions affect phobic experience?

Phobias are more likely to occur in the setting of an easily aroused nervous system. Anxiety and depression can create a hypervigilant, irritable nervous system that increases vulnerability to the development of a phobic disorder. Take the case of George, who suffers from a fear of automobile travel. Treatment in his case would definitely be influenced by his revelation of a past history of panic disorder. His high level of stress would likely cause this anxiety disorder to resurface, and George would be having random and unpredictable panic attacks, perhaps even while sound asleep. Similarly, George's treatment would be influenced by a serious depression in his early 20s, when he found himself unable to get out of bed for a period of weeks. Either scenario would greatly complicate his condition, making the prognosis for complete recovery less promising.

Fortunately, we have effective medical treatments for these problems, and in George's case early recognition and treatment would be an essential component to his successful recovery. This chapter introduces you to the most common anxiety and depression disorders. In any program to address phobias, these underlying emotional illnesses must be dealt with first and treated medically if indicated.

ASSESSING VULNERABILITY TO PHOBIC DISORDERS

Environmental and genetic factors make each of our minds unique. Specific emotional illnesses are not directly inherited, only the vulnerability for these disorders. Whether or not we develop them depends on environmental factors.

Leading genetic research has concluded that genes rank behind stress in causing depression and anxiety. Yet genetics definitely plays a role in vulnerability, as can be seen from twin studies. The influence of genetics can also be seen in the fact that family members tend to respond well to the same medical regimen. We're born with certain genetic predispositions and with a fundamental temperament and personality type. There is no simple "one bad gene" explanation for phobic vulnerability, as in Huntington's disease, sickle-cell anemia, or cystic fibrosis. As with coronary artery disease, hypertension, and diabetes, we feel multiple genes make small contributions to overall vulnerability.

Environmental Factors

Multiple environmental factors increase or decrease our vulnerability to phobias of all kinds:

- Parenting and early life experiences.
- Stress of adolescence, college, marriage, job, and finances.
- Toxins, drugs, alcohol, and stimulants.
- Illness and disease.
- Medications.
- Social support.
- Coping skills.

Some of these experiences, such as childhood abuse and neglect, are largely beyond our control. Other stresses are directly caused by our attitude and choices. The "two hit hypothesis" asserts that we need a one–two punch from genetics and the environment to develop depression or anxiety disorders.

Temperament and personality are leading factors in predicting vulnerability. Temperament is our disposition at birth, and therefore genetically determined. The four basic temperaments are timid, bold, cheerful, and melancholic.

About 15 to 20 percent of children are born timid, with more responsive neurologic circuitry that is aroused by even mild stress. As infants, they are more finicky about new foods, shy around strangers, and reluctant to explore new situations. As children, they shrink from social situations and find themselves less popular than other students. As adults, they view new people and situations as potential threats and are uncomfortable where they may be subject to critical scrutiny. Neurochemically, timidity centers on an amygdala that is easily aroused, predisposing the individual to an exaggerated fear response and a higher rate of anxiety disorders than other temperaments.

About 40 percent of us are born with a bold temperament. It is difficult to activate the amygdala of a bold individual. They are less easily frightened, more outgoing, and more eager to interact socially. This makes them popular and builds self-esteem, people skills, and a sense that the world is a positive place where anything is possible.

Those born cheerful are naturally easygoing and upbeat. They are hard to rile and fun to be with. They enjoy life and share their joy naturally and often with others. They have been found to have higher levels of activity in the left frontal lobe of the brain. Those with cheerful temperaments bounce back faster after setbacks and find the positive in any situation. They have a lower lifetime risk of emotional disorders, especially depression.

Those with melancholic temperaments have higher activity in the right frontal lobe. They cannot seem to turn off their pessimism about themselves, others, and life in general. They are prone to moodiness and seem to get hung up on minor problems. Babies who cry more when their mothers leave the room have more activity in their right frontal lobes, while those that don't have more activity on the left side.

Personality type is determined by genetic traits, temperament, parenting, social relations, traumatic experiences, and other environmental stressors. Those who are neurotic, paranoid, histrionic, or avoidant are often too worried about what might go wrong that they can't enjoy what is going right. Because they make others uncomfortable, those with personality disorders often find themselves avoided and isolated. Their relationships crack under self-manufactured stress, as they become their own worst enemy. The personality disorders most susceptible to anxiety and depression are: paranoid, schizoid, compulsive, histrionic, schizotypical, narcissistic, avoidant, dependent, passive-aggressive, antisocial, and borderline.

RECOGNIZING DEPRESSION UNDERLYING PHOBIAS

One of many helpful mnemonics used to help diagnose depression is APES SWIM. The first four letters, APES, pertain to physical symptoms:

A: Appetite reduction or increase (and/or weight).

P: Psychomotor retardation or agitation.

E: Energy reduction (fatigue).

S: Sleep reduction or increase (insomnia or hypersomnia).

The last four letters pertain to psychological symptoms:

S: Suicidal ideation or thoughts of death.

W: Worthlessness or feelings of guilt.

I: Interest lost in activities that used to bring pleasure.

M: Mental ability diminution (difficulty thinking, concentrating, or deciding).

It is estimated that only 40 percent of those with serious, clinical depression ever seek professional help. Perhaps the biggest psychiatric problem of modern times is massive denial. Anxiety is a more common symptom with depression than is depressed mood, or feeling sad. So a patient may not understand why their doctor is prescribing an "antidepressant" when they are just "nervous and stressed."

DIAGNOSES OF DEPRESSION

In assessing the type of depression besetting a patient, the doctor will consider the nature, duration, and intensity of the patient's symptoms. Diagnoses of major depression, unipolar major depression, dysthymic disorder, minor depression, bipolar depression, and seasonal affective disorder are all possibilities.

Major Depression

In major depression, the patient experiences a markedly depressed mood accompanied by many of the previously mentioned symptoms. Anxiety is often associated with major depression, as the person worries if they will get better or if something is drastically wrong within them. Severe symptoms must last at least two weeks, according to diagnostic criteria, and social and work performance significantly impaired. Some patients will describe feelings of "deep sadness," "hopelessness," "numbness," and being "dead inside." They speak with slow voices and downcast eyes. Others may become irritable, restless, or even angry, unable to relax, eat, or sleep. They may have agitated patterns of speaking and moving, with wringing of their hands a common feature.

Unipolar Major Depression

The patient must have experienced one or more major depressive episodes, but no manic episodes (see page 124).

Dysthymic Disorder

The diagnostic features are depressed mood for most of the day, more days than not, over a period of at least two years, with no episodes of major depression during this time. Common symptoms involve disruption of sleeping and eating habits, poor energy, low self-esteem, poor concentration, and difficulty making decisions. Many are self-critical, viewing themselves as boring or ineffective,

Minor Depression

Depressed mood is not necessary to make a diagnosis of depression. In fact, in those with minor depression, the most common complaints are insomnia, fatigue, thoughts of death, and difficulty concentrating. Mild forms of depression cause a greater toll on society because it affects more people and is less likely to be identified and treated than major depression. In fact, those having minor depression without depressed mood account for twice as many days of lost work than those with major depression with depressed mood. Dr. Louis Judd of the National Institute of Mental Health labels this "subsyndromal symptomatic depression," and says it befalls four times the number who meet the full definition of depression.

Seasonal Affective Disorder

Seasonal affective disorder is most common in women and is thought to be caused by a dysfunction of circadian rhythms occurring in the winter because of decreased exposure to full-spectrum light. Prevalence increases as one moves farther from the equator.

Bipolar Depression

In these disorders, the patient experiences periodic and often dramatic mood swings from times of severe melancholy to times of hyperexcitement, called "mania."

Mania: Mania can be either euphoric ("the world is a wonderful place full of love and energy and opportunity") to dysphoric ("the world is an irritable place full of jerks and incompetent people that get in my way"). In either case, the manic patient feels a great amount of energy, needs much less sleep than usual, and often has delusions about his or her abilities and importance. During severe manic episodes, spousal or child abuse is common. Patients with bipolar illness generally spend much less time in their manic phases than their depressive phases. Moving between the two poles of mania and depression is called "cycling." Ninety percent of those who have a single episode of mania will have future recurrences. A manic episode is defined as an elevated, expansive, or irritable mood of at least one week's duration causing significant impairment or hospitalization.

Hypomania: Hypomanic episodes are less severe elevated, expansive, or irritable moods lasting at least four days, with changes observed by others close to the person. It should be noted that many patients feel good during their manic or hypomanic phases: they feel nothing is wrong with them; everybody else has the problem; everybody else is jealous of their powers, success, sexual magnetism, etc. These patients do not seek out the doctor's help during their manic spells—only when they drop into the hole of depression and want to get back to mania again. For diagnosing a hypomanic episode, the patient must have three or more of the following:

1. Inflated self-esteem/delusions of grandeur.
2. Decreased need for sleep.
3. More talkative than usual.
4. Racing thoughts and flights of ideas.
5. Easily distracted.
6. Increase in goal-oriented activity in social life, work, or school.
7. Excessive involvement in high-pleasure/high-risk activities. (Overly expensive shopping, gambling, bungee jumping, sexual indiscretions, etc.)

Bipolar I Disorder: This more severe diagnosis requires that the patient has had a least one true manic episode or mixed episode (met the criteria for manic episode and major depressive episode).

Bipolar II Disorder: This less severe diagnosis is often missed, and requires at least one hypomanic episode and one major depression episode. Because these patients only see the doctor during depression, they are often only treated with antidepressants and don't get better because the hypomania is not treated first with mood stabilizers.

Cyclothymic Disorder: Symptoms of both manic and depressive disorders are present, but only to a minimal degree. Mood changes fluctuate from despair to elation, but never qualify for a major depressive episode or a manic or hypomanic episode. The person is labeled as temperamental, moody, unpredictable, and unreliable. Problems and misunderstandings are common in the person's work and social life. Cyclothymic disorder often overlaps with borderline personality disorder, where the person experiences instability in personal relationships, poor self-image, fears of separation and abandonment, and excessive anger/inflexibility when plans change.

RECOGNIZING ANXIETY AS A CONDITION UNDERLYING PHOBIAS

Studies have shown that 20 to 30 percent of patients in a general medical practice suffer from clinically significant anxiety. Because of chemical changes that occur during the grief reaction, anxiety becomes more likely. Usually, our brain has a balance of chemical and neurological interaction, which is much like the blinders on a horse, keeping us from seeing all the snakes in the road. Life is, by its nature, insecure and uncertain. Loss strips away the false sense of security and control and makes us look at the anxiety-provoking reality. If someone already was suffering from an anxiety disorder, they will be especially vulnerable to relapse at this time.

Normal Anxiety: "Normal" anxiety involves accurate timing and proportion in response to stress. A bumpy airplane ride, public speaking, near-miss accident, or important examination may all trigger a mild anxiety response with an increased heart rate, shakiness, or a cold sweat.

Clinical Anxiety: In clinically significant anxiety, symptoms appear frequently and out of proportion to stimuli. These symptoms then interfere with the usual patterns and habits of the person's life, such as work, sexual function, sleep, and appetite.

GAD

Generalized anxiety disorder (GAD) is the most common of the anxiety disorders.

Predisposing Factors: Relatives with anxiety disorders, shyness, social inhibition, history of vivid childhood fears.

Symptoms: Symptoms of the mind include uncontrolled worry, restlessness, irritability, apprehension, insomnia, and problems concentrating. Symptoms of the body include chest pain (33 percent), abdominal pain (31 percent), headache (28 percent), and fatigue/exhaustion (26 percent).

Diagnosis: Persistent anxiety and worry, more days than not, during the past 6 months. Must exclude other anxiety disorders, medication reactions, or medical conditions (such as cardiac arrhythmia or overactive thyroid).

Other Features: Pessimism, substance abuse (alcohol, sedatives, sleeping pills). Of those with GAD, 80 percent will develop depression and social phobia.

PANIC DISORDER

Predisposing Factors: If you have a parent with panic disorder, you have a four to seven times greater chance of developing this disorder. Starts in young adulthood. Onset after age 45 is rare.

Symptoms and Diagnosis: Unlike anxiety attacks, which occur with an identifiable stimulus (specific phobia, excessive worry), panic attacks are unpredictable and recurrent. A panic attack may wake you from sleep. The American Psychiatric Association uses the following criteria for diagnosis:

Four or more of the following must be abruptly and intensely present and peak within 10 minutes: palpitations, sweating, shakiness, shortness of breath, feeling of choking, chest pain or discomfort, nausea or abdominal pain, feeling faint or dizzy, chills or hot flashes, numbness and tingling, fear of losing control or going crazy, fear of doom or impending death, or derealization or depersonalization (feeling of unreality or being detached from oneself).

Other Features: Self-medication is common (alcohol and benzodiazepines most common), as well as frequent visits to the ER. More than half develop major depression, prone to co-existing anxiety disorders (agoraphobia in 30 percent, social phobia in 20 percent, GAD in 25 percent, specific phobia in 10 to 20 percent).

OTHER ANXIETY DISORDERS

Acute Stress Disorder: Clinically significant anxiety symptoms occur after a traumatic experience (for example, car accident, assault, or witness of violent crime). Acute stress disorders usually resolve within eight weeks of the traumatic incident.

Post-Traumatic Stress Disorder (PTSD): Recurrent anxiety that lasts longer than eight weeks is a feature of post-traumatic stress disorder. The degree of anxiety corresponds to the proximity of the victim to the traumatic event. Common traumas causing PTSD include violent personal assault, rape, hostage situations, torture, war, serious accidents, surviving the death of a loved one, and being diagnosed with a life-threatening illness. The recurrent anxiety symptoms cause significant distress and impairment in occupational and social functioning.

Obsessive-Compulsive Disorder (OCD): In this disorder, the sufferer develops repeated and ritualistic behaviors in an attempt to control or chase away the obsessive thoughts and anxieties. Checking and rechecking doors, windows, and stoves, washing the hands dozens of times a day, needing to have things in a particular order or arrangement are all examples of obsessive-compulsive behavior. Those with OCD wish they could stop the recurring thoughts and images that lead to their often bizarre behavior. But when they try to quit their rituals, the anxiety commonly increases.

Anorexia Nervosa/Bulimia: Anxiety about gaining weight causes an unhealthy relationship with food. Anorexics suffer from self-induced malnutrition because of this fear. Bulimics try to gain control over their intake of food by gorging themselves and then purging their meal through self-induced vomiting.

Hypochondriasis: This is the unwarranted fear of having a serious illness. Amorphous fears are transferred to a part of the body that can be "blamed." The patient then seeks to heal and repair the problem. After seeking professional evaluation, multiple tests, and a large amount of reassurance, the patient may then imagine a different part of the body is unwell. We tend to mock the hypochondriac, while we afford more sympathy to those with other anxiety disorders, such as panic disorder.

Trichotillomania: Disorder characterized by pulling out one's own hair, particularly in stressful situations.

Body Dysmorphic Disorder: Interestingly, this is a variant of obsessive-compulsive disorder, where the afflicted obsesses about some part of their body that they perceive as ugly (typically nose, chin lips, breasts, fingers, legs, or sexual organs). These patients commonly end up seeing multiple plastic surgeons, believing that they will feel better once the imagined deformity is corrected. Unfortunately, because the underlying problem is really an anxiety disorder, these patients do not find relief even after multiple procedures. Michael Jackson's many apparent surgical procedures may be a case in point.

Depressive Syndromes Related to Hormonal Imbalances: Premenstrual dysphoric disorder, postpartum depression, peri- and postmenopausal mood changes are all well documented. SSRIs seem particularly effective here. Prozac, marketed as Sarafem, has been approved for use just when needed on days of PMS-triggered mood changes.

Chapter 7

MEDICAL EVALUATION AND TREATMENT OF PHOBIAS

This chapter answers three questions:

1. How can we predict which people are likely to develop phobias?
2. What steps are recommended in a thorough medical evaluation for phobic symptoms?
3. What medications are commonly prescribed for the treatment of anxiety and phobias?

It is relatively easy to predict who among us is most likely to develop a phobia. Those with a family history of anxiety or phobias, those exposed to abuse, neglect, or poor parenting strategies in childhood, those who experimented with drugs or were previously diagnosed with a personality disorder or emotional illness, and those who experienced a deep trauma or are dealing with excessive life stressors are especially vulnerable. Health conditions such as hormonal changes seen in adolescence and perimenopause, thyroid disorders, chronic pain, chronic fatigue, malignancies, and many other ailments strongly affect us emotionally and can drain our neurochemistry. Eating and sleeping disorders can be the cause or consequence of anxiety, and one dysfunction will often lead to another in a downward spiral of increasing anxiety and nervous system aggravation.

For all these reasons, you will want and need a full medical assessment to rule out other health problems that might be contributing to your phobia problem. Anyone who suffers from phobias deserves a complete physical from a primary care doctor, as well as an evaluation by a psychiatrist, psychologist, or therapist. Your primary doctor may or may not feel comfortable treating phobias or emotional disorders medically. Before undertaking medical treatment, you may want to seek the expert opinion of a psychiatrist. Certainly you should feel at ease about asking if some treatment you have read about in these pages or on the Internet is appropriate for you. Also be sure to discuss a remedy that worked for a family member with a similar problem.

AN EXAMPLE OF MEDICAL EVALUATION IN THE TREATMENT OF PHOBIAS

Peggy is a woman in her mid-40s who is happily married with two well-behaved teenagers. She is cheerful and outgoing by nature, and is known for her extensive volunteer work in the community. It came as a surprise, therefore, when she confided to her doctor that she had developed a great discomfort and anxiety in social situations. She would make any excuse to avoid speaking in public and was begging off on the fundraisers and charity events she had previously organized and planned. On further questioning, it turned out she had been under a lot of stress. First were the financial worries that the family business was failing and would need to be sold. There had also been an illness with her mother-in-law and the death of the cherished family dog. Things started going downhill when she developed insomnia, lying awake for hours at night trying to figure out how the bills would be paid and whether her husband would find a new career or business. She would wake up in a sweat with her heart racing and her hands shaking with anxiety and panic. She then began having these attacks randomly at charitable functions, and would have to excuse herself.

Peggy felt old friends were beginning to whisper behind her back and was afraid she would have an attack in front of community members and humiliate herself. Sleep became more difficult, and she lost her appetite. In this case, real-life stressors led to a sleep disorder, and eventually an eating disorder. The neurochemical imbalances caused by unrelenting worry and sleep deprivation then led to panic disorder. Fear of a symptom attack caused phobic avoidance of social situations, which is an agoraphobic response rather than true social phobia. Peggy was treated immediately with a drug to correct the chemical imbalance of panic disorder (Zoloft), in combination with the anxiolytic Klonopin, which works immediately to improve sleep and block anxiety attacks. She felt better the next morning, and her symptoms were resolved in two weeks. This quick success is due in part to Peggy's lack of any previous health or anxiety conditions, her strong sense of self-worth, and the great deal of love and support she drew from family and friends. Winning the lottery would probably have also worked, or any substantial resolution of her financial worries, but medical intervention was appropriate and greatly limited her suffering, preventing further embarrassment to her reputation or loss of her ability to function as a mom and wife.

The choice of medical tools must be tailored to each individual situation. Your doctor or psychiatrist will need to know everything about you to make the proper decisions in this regard. This chapter merely familiarizes you with the many pharmaceuticals we have in our arsenal to support your recovery as quickly as possible.

THE MEDICAL EVALUATION

The following is a summary of the different "spheres of sensitivity" that contribute to our vulnerability to have an imbalanced nervous system just ripe for the development of a phobia. In our clinic, we evaluate each of these areas of a patient's life to find ways to help bring their system back into balance. This will make their road to recovery from phobias much easier, and with a significantly higher success rate.

This is a diagram of interlocking spheres with the following labels:

Sphere 1: Life Experiences (parenting, trauma, work/relationship/ financial stressors, etc.)

Sphere 2: Personality Disorders (borderline, narcissistic, dependent, avoidant, paranoid, etc.)

Sphere 3: Emotional Disorders (including mood disorders, anxiety disorders, and behavioral disorders and their genetic components).

Sphere 4: Medical Conditions (hormonal changes, diabetes, heart disease, thyroid and other endocrine problems, migraines, autoimmune diseases, chronic pain, etc.)

Sphere 5: Dysfunctional Activities and Addictions (including substance abuse, spending money irresponsibly, gambling, overworking, sexual obsessions, and some hobbies).

Sphere 6: Lack of Support and Poor Coping Skills and Strategies.

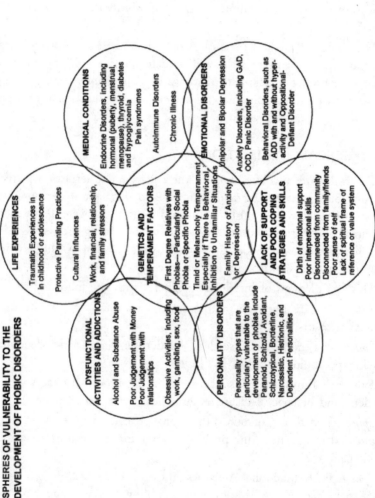

Gardner and Bell, 2004

Sphere 7: Genetic and Temperament Factors (such as family history of anxiety and phobias; timid or melancholy temperaments—especially with an aspect of behavioral inhibition to new and unfamiliar situations).

WHAT TO EXPECT IN A MEDICAL EVALUATION

Getting a medical evaluation is fairly standard, routine, and straight-forward. Dr. Gardner's clinic performs this service in two stages, called (unoriginally) the first half and the second half exams. In the first half, the focus is on your history. This includes your personal history and habits, such as what you do for a living; your marital status; your education; whether you drink, smoke, or use recreational drugs; and so on. You may be asked to fill out some short questionnaires designed to elicit any underlying emotional disorders. Then we focus on your medical history, including previous medical problems, medications, allergies, surgeries, and health problems in your family. Then a "review of systems" is performed, which is a list of questions about all your bodily functions and complaints. With all this information, we make a "problem list," which is a compilation of your known or previously diagnosed conditions, as well as your undiagnosed complaints. From this list we then tailor a plan to most effectively get the answers we need. The plan may include getting blood work, an x-ray of your chest, a sample of your urine, and an electrocardiogram of your heart for starters. If indicated, the evaluation may include a more in-depth look at the heart with the treadmill stress test, heart CT scan, 24-hour heart monitor, or echocardiogram tests.

Sometimes a look at the brain is helpful. This is usually best accomplished by MRI scans to look at the structure of the brain. Other brain scans, known as SPECT scans, can give information on brain metabolism and function. Relating to phobias, some of the important labs and tests your physician may order include:

- ⮞ Thyroid function tests (looking for high or low thyroid performance).
- ⮞ Fasting glucose (looking for low blood sugar, or hypoglycemia).
- ⮞ Calcium level (looking for an overactive parathyroid gland causing high calcium levels).
- ⮞ Cardiac enzyme tests (especially if you have chest pains and heart palpitations).

- ~ Drug screen (if illicit drug use is suspected; your physician will ask your permission for this).

- ~ A 24-hour urine for 5-hydroxyindoleacetic acid (5-HIAA) levels (looking for an internal tumor that secretes stress hormones called pheochromocytoma).

- ~ Head CT scan (this is a computerized 3-D x-ray designed to identify any structural abnormalities in your brain).

- ~ MRI scan (instead of radiation, this scan uses nonionizing electromagnetic energy to image the brain and spinal cord).

- ~ Echocardiogram (uses sound waves to produce an image of the heart structures, especially looking for mitral valve prolapse, a condition that can cause heart palpitations).

- ~ ECG or 24-hour holter monitor (to exclude heart damage or arrhythmias).

- ~ Provocative studies with carbon dioxide, sodium lactate, or yohimbine, as well as positron emission tomography (PET) studies are largely reserved for research purposes at this point.

When all the tests are completed and results received at the office, we then do the second half. Here we go over all your results and give you copies for your personal file. Then the physician does a routine physical exam appropriate for your age and complaints. After all this is done, a new "problem list" is generated, adding on new findings from the tests and physical exam, if any. Finally, a specialist may be called in to give an opinion on a specific question. This might be a neurologist, cardiologist, psychiatrist, endocrinologist, or any number of other physicians with special insight and expertise. Often, no other special tests or specialty consults are necessary, and we are ready to decide on a treatment plan for medical intervention.

MEDICAL TREATMENT OF ANXIETY AND PHOBIAS

Before tackling the treatment of your anxiety or phobia, your physician will want to get all medical problems identified and properly stabilized or corrected. Because they are known to cause anxiety, several conditions should be controlled as soon as possible. This includes diabetes; hypoglycemia; thyroid disorders; heart conditions, including arrhythmias and coronary artery disease; drug or alcohol overuse, headache or other pain syndromes; autoimmune disorders, including fibromyalgia; sleep disorders; hormonal and other endocrine imbalances; and annoying digestive problems such as acid reflux and irritable bowel disorder. This can often be accomplished concurrently with the initiation of medical treatment for anxiety. Also remember that other emotional conditions often coexist with anxiety and phobias, especially depression. These must be recognized and treated as well. Most anxieties and phobias, if the severity of symptoms and resulting dysfunction warrants it, can be significantly improved with modern medications that can be prescribed by your primary care doctor or psychiatrist. For many, these medications may well give the first real relief and sense of hope that the patient has felt in years. If your doctor feels medication is warranted, don't hesitate to give it a try. You can always come off the medication if you don't like it.

How Will Your Doctor Choose the Right Medication for You?

Even the best psychiatrist in the world may need some time to find the right medical regimen for you, if that is what you need. Often, the "trial-and-error" method is used, as there is no magical diagnostic tool that can see exactly what's going on in your brain. In the expected case that the doctor gets the diagnosis right, you may have to try several drugs before finding the one that works best with your system. The process of finding the right medication is greatly helped by an accurate history and diagnosis. You are more likely to respond favorably to a particular medication if a close family member tolerated it well and got good results.

Dr. Gardner's clinic has found that many individuals have a variety of diagnoses that overlap. For instance, it is not uncommon for a patient to have social phobia, panic disorder, unipolar depression, and attention deficit disorder all at the same time. How can we make the most simple and effective treatment plan to cover all the bases?

Understanding how the brain responds to the different neurotransmitters that we can manipulate and augment through medical intervention, we have a rational and scientific method of determining a program that is likely to work for you. This way of addressing emotional disorders has been advocated by the preeminent neurobiologist Dr. Stephen Stahl. The detailed and thoughtful paradigm that we follow for determining the medical regimen that will best address your symptoms is a constant work in progress, and has been largely the brainchild of Dr. Brent Cox, M.D., a respected psychiatrist, teacher, and lecturer in the San Francisco Bay Area.

Following is a summary and simplification of this model:

Symptomatic features that respond to SEROTONIN *augmentation:*

1. Significant obsessional ruminations and fears or behavioral compulsions.

2. The tendency to catastrophize with a high level of sensitivity to perceived external threats.

3. Carbohydrate cravings or binge-eating patterns, where the patient uses food to help stabilize their mood.

4. Intense irritability or episodic rage attacks (road rage).

5. Anxiety and anxiety attacks due to underlying anxiety disorders, including OCD, panic disorder, post-traumatic stress disorder, generalized anxiety disorder, and body dysmorphic disorder.

6. Depressive mood of seasonal affective disorder and hormonal fluctuations (seen after childbirth, before the menstrual period, and during the perimenopausal change of life).

7. For eating disorders such as bulimia or binge eating (specifically high doses of Prozac and Celexa).

8. Found to be beneficial in treating the symptoms of fibromyalgia syndrome, chronic fatigue syndrome, and migraine headaches.

Drugs with serotonin activity include Prozac, Paxil, Zoloft, Celexa, Luvox, Lexapro, Anafranil, Serzone, Effexor, Remeron, Elavil, Sinequan, and Cymbalta.

Symptomatic features that respond to NOREPINEPHRINE *augmentation:*

1. Impairments in attention and concentration.

2. Slowness in information processing and deficiencies in working memory.

3. Psychomotor retardation (slowing of physical movement and response).

4. Diminished energy and easy fatigability.

5. Melancholic depression.

6. Bipolar depression.

7. Difficult, treatment-resistant depression.

8. Cognitive symptoms of attention deficit disorder.

9. Binge eating (specifically Wellbutrin).

10. Chronic pain syndromes (specifically Effexor and Remeron).

11. Hot flashes of perimenopause (specifically Effexor).

Drugs with norepinephrine activity include Effexor, Wellbutrin, Remeron, Strattera, Desipramine, and Nortryptiline.

Symptomatic features that respond to DOPAMINE *augmentation:*

1. Diminished capacity to experience pleasure and excitement (losing interest in sex, hobbies, and spontaneous fun).

2. Impairments in attention and concentration.

3. Diminished volitional capabilities, as well as low motivation and initiative.

4. Decreased energy and increased fatigability.

5. Diminished libido and sexual responsiveness.

6. Atypical and bipolar depression (specifically Wellbutrin and Parnate).

7. Cognitive impairments of attention deficit disorder.

8. Addictive behaviors involving nicotine, alcohol, opioids, marijuana, as well as risk-taking behavior (compulsive gambling, for example).

9. Helpful in obesity and chronic pain syndromes.

Drugs with dopamine activity include Wellbutrin, Parnate, Effexor (high dose), Zoloft (high dose), Dexedrine, and Mirapex

Symptomatic features that respond to MOOD STABILIZERS *and* ATYPICAL ANTIPSYCHOTICS:

Terms such as "mood stabilizers" and "antipsychotics" are somewhat frightening to readers and may seem to have no place in a book about phobias. The drugs in this category do treat the more serious psychiatric conditions of bipolar mania, psychosis, and schizophrenia, and have been approved by the FDA for these purposes. However, as is true of many medications, these drugs have other "off-label" uses. This means that doctors have found them to be very beneficial in other circumstances for which they have not been formally approved. In the case of mood stabilizers and atypical antipsychotics, we have found great benefit in quieting the irritable, hypersensitive, and hypervigilant nervous systems that are often fertile grounds for anxiety and phobic disorders. These types of drugs have been extremely helpful in controlling the following symptoms:

1. Poor sleep architecture or not achieving restful sleep.

2. Nighttime and early morning anxiety attacks.

3. Excessive rumination (thinking about the same thing over and over) and racing of the mind (not able to slow down your thoughts).

4. Feeling of "too much energy" seen in bipolar manic patients.

5. Excessive paranoid ideation (thinking others are scrutinizing you in a negative way or are "out to get you").

6. Anger and oppositional behavior.

7. General chronic anxiety or nervousness.

Drugs that are in the family of mood stabilizers and atypical antipsychotics include Risperdal, Seroquel, Zyprexa, Abilify, Geodone, Lamictal, Depakote, Lithium, Neurontin, Topamax, and Keppra.

Symptomatic features that respond to BENZODIAZEPINES:

Recall the GABA neuronal system we learned about earlier when exploring the physiology of fear. This system suppresses neuronal excitement throughout the brain. Benzodiazepines stimulate GABA receptors, thereby triggering the relaxation response both psychologically and physically. Well it seems like a "no-brainer" that these drugs would be the mainstay of therapy for anxiety and phobias. Unfortunately, they have the potential for overuse and addiction, and are potentially fatal in overdose. Because many anxious patients are also depressed, this is a real concern. Benzodiazepines are all related to Valium, and have been modified to change how quickly they work (time to peak blood concentration) and quickly they wear off (half-life of the drug). Some benzodiazepines last a few hours, while others last a whole day. The symptoms we would expect to improve with this class are:

1. Poor sleep patterns.

2. Anxiety and panic attacks.

3. Phobic anxiety (occasional, situational use).

4. Muscle spasms and reducing the brain's vulnerability to seizure.

5. Quick relief of irritable/aggressive mood.

Drugs that are in the benzodiazepine family include Valium, Xanax, Ativan, Librium, Tranxene, Serax, Xanax XR, and Klonopin. Benzodiazepines that have been designed to work as sleeping pills (quick onset of action and wearing off by eight hours) include Restoril, Halcion, and Dalmane. Other sleeping pills, such as Ambien and Sonata, also work by affecting the GABA system.

Symptomatic features that respond to BETA-BLOCKERS:

One of the oldest treatments for phobias was the use of the short-acting beta-blocker propanolol for those with speaker's nerves, or fear of public speaking. Beta receptors are the places where our stress hormones bind when our sympathetic nervous system wants to prepare the body for the fight or flight response. They are in our muscles, arteries, heart, and glands, and are responsible for the physical fear symptoms of rapid heart rate, tremors, sweats, dizziness, nausea, and just about any other symptom caused by sympathetic nervous system activation. Because beta-blockers bind to beta-receptors throughout the body, this fear response is largely prevented. Taken before a speech or presentation, this drug gives the patient the confidence that they won't embarrass themselves by one of these symptoms. Because beta-blockers are primarily used to control blood pressure and heart rate in cardiac patients, they are especially appropriate for phobia patients who have these medical conditions. In this case, the longer-acting drugs in this category, such as Atenolol, would be more appropriate.

USING THE SYMPTOM-BASED APPROACH TO TREATMENT OF PHOBIAS

You may recall the example of Paul from Chapter 5. He came to our clinic asking for medical treatment of OCD. His fear of germs with excessive washing and cleaning had caused problems with his social and work life. He had turned inward to embrace alcohol and isolation. But things just got worse, with difficulty sleeping, early awakening with anxiety attacks, depressed mood with loss of passion and enjoyment in life, and a loss of motivation with difficulty focusing and concentrating on the task at hand. The many possible diagnoses that could be entertained here have overlapping features and symptoms. Besides his OCD, he is exhibiting features of unipolar depression, panic disorder, ADD, substance abuse, and a sleep disorder.

To treat Paul successfully, we don't have to unwind this tangled ball of string. We just need to listen to his symptoms. Many of these symptoms we recognize right away as being influenced by the serotonin neurotrans-mitter pathways, namely anxiety and anxiety attacks, depressed mood, and obsessional ruminations with behavioral compulsions. In addition, many of his symptoms would be addressed by augmenting his norepi-nephrine pathways, in particular his impairments in attention and concen-tration, diminished energy and fatigue, and depression. Finally, enhancing dopamine would also be of benefit, not just in improving his energy, mood, and attention, but also in addressing his low motivation, lack of passion and sense of pleasure, and helping curb his desire for alcohol.

Feeling that the alcohol overuse and sleep problems were secondary and would clear up after treating the anxiety and depression features, Dr. Gardner chose to start with the serotonin drug Lexapro and the dopamine and nore-pinephrine drug Wellbutrin. After a week on 5mg of Lexapro, he was in-creased to 10mg. Wellbutrin XL 150mg was started at the same time, both medications taken together in the morning. He was offered Antabuse, a drug that causes nausea and vomiting if you drink alcohol, but he decided he could stop the alcohol on his own. Two weeks later, Paul felt 50 percent better as far as his OCD symptoms were concerned. In addition, depressive feelings of despair had lifted completely. He had no side effects to either drug and had completely stopped his alcohol habit. Two weeks after that, Paul was sensing some continued improvement in his OCD symptoms of washing and cleaning, but still experienced anxiety during the workday and at night. He had some improvement in motivation and energy, and was doing better at work. To treat the anxiety more aggressively, we increased the Lexapro to 15mg. On the sixth week after starting treatment, Paul was sig-nificantly improved, with anxiety symptoms 80 to 90 pecent under control, no awakening with anxiety, no depression, no alcohol use, and reasonably good concentration, motivation, and energy. His hand washing had dropped from 40 times a day to less than 10 times.

If he were still having poor sleep patterns and awakening with anxiety, we would have considered adding a low-dose atypical antipsychotic such as Risperdal or a benzopdiazepine such as Klonopin at bedtime. Certain ingrained thoughts and behaviors die hard, however, and Paul was sent back to cognitive behavioral therapy, which has reduced his ritualistic clean-ing behaviors. Because obsessive washing was his coping strategy and main tool to calm his anxious nerves, the process of letting go involved replacing old behaviors with new, more functional, learned strategies. In this way,

Paul took an old, dysfunctional tool from his toolbox and replaced it with the right tool to succeed in the job of life.

AN EXAMPLE OF MEDICAL TREATMENT FOR MULTIPLE UNDERLYING CONDITIONS

Jason is a 17-year-old high school dropout with a criminal record for drug dealing and armed robbery. He grew up in a middle-class neighborhood with his mother, father, and grandmother. His mother had problems with drug and alcohol, and his father traveled a lot, so he was mostly raised by his grandmother. He was sent to school psychologists in elementary school for his disruptive behavior in the classroom. He routinely was at the bottom of his class, and didn't seem to care. Whenever his father came home, he could expect angry lectures about his poor performance and bad attitude. These sessions would often lead to violence and a beating. Jason left home at age 14 to live in the garage of an older friend who was also doing poorly in school and was selling drugs. Eventually Jason was arrested and spent two years in a juvenile facility.

Before being released, the judge had required a medical and psychological evaluation. During this evaluation, it was found that Jason had a fear of falling asleep, and was nodding off just a few hours a day. He had chronic headaches and was known for his short temper and severe anger flares that would get him into fights at the correction facility. His list of disciplinary setbacks was long and extensive. He had an odd habit of cutting himself with any available sharp object to induce pain and bleeding, and had numerous scars on his inner arms. He would also need to check doors and locks several times before he was convinced that his room was safe. This fear of sleeping started one night in the juvenile correction facility when a male guard had entered his room at night and slipped into bed with him. Jason had awakened startled to find the guard touching him in his private area. A frightened shout made the guard quickly leave after warning him to "keep his mouth shut." It never happened again, but Jason was petrified it would, and often awoke from sleep with an anxiety attack. He soon found he could not fall asleep, was getting severe headaches, and had no tolerance for confrontation. His anger problems made him too volatile to release back to the care of his parents or some "halfway house," and the judge was considering extending his incarceration for "bad behavior."

In this case, it is easy to see that a traumatic experience of sexual molestation led to deep anxiety that manifested itself in behaviors that are consistent with obsessive-compulsive disorder. Cutting the skin is done by anxious individuals to distract themselves from their fears, and obsessive checking of door locks is another behavior typical of the hypervigilant state of the OCD patient. In addition, he had a history of childhood attention deficit hyperactivity disorder (ADHD) that had led to poor performance in school. Instead of getting help and support from his family and the school, he was punished, beaten, and labeled as a "problem child" with a "bad attitude." His anger first grew out of frustration of his behavior and learning disorder (ADHD), but was later directed toward abusive and dysfunctional parents and authority figures in general. Jason hated himself. He could not list a single thing he enjoyed, was good at, or had accomplished. His anger at himself and the world could be seen in his slouching posture, angry and violent tattoos and piercings, and sullen gaze. He looked 10 years older due to the lack of sleep and pain of his chronic headaches.

On the first visit with Jason, we started him on Risperdal at bedtime and Strattera in the morning, and arranged for regular psychotherapy to include cognitive behavioral therapy (CBT) for his OCD. The reason for the choice of the atypical antipsychotic Risperdal was to gain quick control of his sleeping patterns and to stop the nighttime anxiety. This class of medications helps to blunt the anger response. His headaches were thought to be due to sleep deprivation, and would resolve with restoration of deep restorative sleep. It could have been argued that we should have started a serotonin drug at the same time for his OCD symptoms, but we felt his serotonin would restore itself naturally with a period of good sleep. Remember that Jason's OCD was not apparent until after the stressful experience that triggered anxiety and sleep problems. He did not seem to have an underlying strong genetic predisposition to this disorder. On the other hand, he did have a long history of undiagnosed ADHD, which we elected to treat with Strattera.

The benefit of this intervention, along with the CBT, was evident within weeks. The headaches resolved, he was no longer confrontational, he was sleeping six hours a night with no breakthrough anxiety attacks, and he no longer feared going to sleep, as long as he had his medication. He has seen a great improvement in mental focus and concentration, and has enrolled in a vocational training program offered by the state department of corrections. The entire focus of anger, anxiety, worthlessness, and negativity was changed to a hopeful, cooperative, and positive attitude because of the professional intervention and support he finally received. After family counseling, it was decided that Jason would be released to live with his parents during his probationary period, rather than spend an extra year in jail. A potentially serious threat and liability to society now has a chance to turn his life around.

A CASE OF MEDICAL DESENSITIZATION

Lisa, a woman in her 40s who had just been offered a job in San Francisco, was about to turn down the position due to a fear of driving over bridges that cross over water. Even the thought of the trip made her queasy and unable to focus or concentrate. The actual sight of a bridge brought on heart palpitations and a feeling she was about to faint. Because she lived in Marin County, any commute to the city involved crossing a major bridge over the bay. Her other alternative, the ferry system, even evoked a stronger fear of the water itself. I asked her to take a quarter milligram of Alprazolam, a short acting anxiolytic medication, one hour before her morning commute. A year later, at her annual checkup, I noted she had never asked for a refill of the medication. I asked her if it had not worked. "No, it worked perfectly," she said, explaining that she needed it less and less as she continued to expose herself to the bridge crossing. "I just started breaking them in half, and then into smaller pieces until I could go over the bridge fine without them." It is felt by many therapists that drugs that block anxiety are counterproductive to exposure therapy. Emotional learning, they feel, would be muted by the drug, thereby making the exposure experience ineffective. By serendipity, we found that small doses of the short-acting benzodiazepines at the initiation of phobic exposure were very helpful and sometimes necessary to start exposure treatment. Doses can often be rapidly diminished and withdrawn, even as the exposure is gradually intensified.

MEDICATION TO HELP SPEED
THE UNLEARNING OF PHOBIAS

You may remember from our earlier discussion of brain function that the amygdala regulates emotions and organizes the fear response. Next door in the hippocampus, memories of fear and trauma are stored, and a feedback loop with the amygdala is created. This feedback loop allows the triggering of the amygdala's anxiety response whenever a trauma is remembered. In this way, fear becomes a swift and primitive reaction that is learned and hardwired into the deep centers of the brain. In fact, it happens so fast and reflexively that the higher rational centers of the brain, like the prefrontal cortex, do not have time to explain and inform the deeper anxiety centers that the fear is unreasonable and the fear reaction should be aborted. This is why trying to talk someone out of their phobias through rational arguments does not work. Desensitization through exposure therapy has been shown to gradually extinguish specific and social phobias. This is because new memories are being created that a feared object or situation is not so bad, after all. When the brain discovers that it can survive the phobia exposure with less and less difficulty, it gradually unlearns the old hippocampal memory that was responsible for triggering the phobic fear response. But exposure therapy is often a long and painful process. What if this process of unlearning could be sped up with a medical intervention? Michael Davis of Emory University has discovered that some proteins in the amygdala called NMDA receptors appear to speed up the process of unlearning fear. His work with rats in the laboratory has lead to a new and unique medical strategy for the treatment of phobias. In describing the role of NMDA receptors, Davis explains: "Many years ago, we discovered that the NMDA receptor protein in the amygdala was not only necessary to learn to be afraid, it was also necessary to learn *not* to be afraid." A drug called D-Cycloserine (DCS) was known to be able to boost the levels of NMDA proteins. It had been used in the past as a treatment for tuberculosis—now it would be tested to see if it could play a new role in speeding up the extinction of fear during exposure therapy. A group of 27 people with acrophobia were given two sessions of virtual reality treatment for their fear of heights. Immediately afterward, three subgroups formed; one was given a placebo (sugar pill), another was given a low dose of DCS, and the third was given a higher dose of DCS. The results were published in the November 2004 issue of *Archives of General Psychiatry.* Those who received the DCS were able to conquer their phobia more effectively than those who received the placebo pill. Even three months later, the DCS groups were still reporting better control over their phobia. The fact that the drug has no side effects and only needs to be used for a short time during the unlearning (exposure) process is especially appealing.

THE ROLE OF PATIENT AND FAMILY EDUCATION

The treating physician's most valuable tool is replacing misinformation, confusion, insecurity, and frustration with clear information and encouragement. The process of education should include the family, concerned friends, and significant others. This is the patient's support group, and they must all understand the diagnosis clearly as well as the rationale for any medical or psychotherapeutic treatment. Family and friends can help by encouraging the patient to confront fears, help with medication and therapy compliance, and learn when to stay out of the way and let the patient venture forth on his own.

MEDICAL EVALUATION AS A FORM OF THERAPY

Occasionally a patient's phobia disappears during the course of the medical evaluation itself, before any pharmacologic therapy is initiated. We often hear a patient say, "I already feel so much better" after just the first visit. We also appreciate the many hurdles they had to overcome just to get to the office and begin to face the problem. Validation, reassurance, and encouragement go a long way in giving an initial sense of relief and release. The experience of seeing or hearing the truth firsthand from the doctor allows a deep form of believing to occur. Being shown or taught that something you thought was a source of worry and concern does not actually exist can often bring about a seemingly miraculous "cure." For many, the reassurance from a thorough and trusted professional can improve symptoms right away. After spending much time in explaining and giving helpful information on anxiety, doctors will often give a short-acting anxiety medication for a few days to give the patient some immediate relief. They are frequently surprised at how often the medication is never even picked up from the pharmacy because the patient felt "so much better" just from coming in and talking about the problem.

FACING THE TRUTH AND FINDING FREEDOM

Lee, an old friend from childhood, called for Dr. Gardner's advice one weekend. He was sure there was something growing in his throat that made swallowing difficult. It started when he had seen a TV special on throat cancer and was made aware of his own risk for this disease from his habit of chewing tobacco. He definitely felt a lump back there, and was afraid it might obstruct his breathing or swallowing at some point. He had no serious symptoms, but got so wound up about it that he could not sleep or think of anything else. Suspecting globus hystericus, an anxiety-based phobic fear that the throat will close off and become obstructed due to an abnormal growth, Dr. Gardner sent Lee for a diagnostic and therapeutic test called the barium swallow. This simple test involves the patient swallowing a liquid that shows up well on the x-ray video technique called fluoroscopy. I specifically instructed the radiologist to let Lee observe the video to see that his throat was completely clear and unobstructed as the fluid passed down to the stomach. At the moment of this observation, all of Lee's symptoms and growing phobic fears resolved immediately. The "lump" he had felt for many anxious days and weeks disappeared from his sensory awareness because it had disappeared from his belief system.

The more concretely we confront a cognitive misperception, the more dramatically and quickly it will lose its hold on our deeply held beliefs.

Chapter 8

THE ROLE OF COUNSELING, PSYCHOTHERAPY, AND COGNITIVE BEHAVIORAL THERAPY IN OVERCOMING PHOBIAS

This chapter answers four questions:

1. What is cognitive behavioral therapy and how can it help recovery from phobias?
2. What are "wrong thoughts," and how can they be replaced by positive messages?
3. What is exposure therapy as it applies to the treatment of phobias?
4. How can counseling address stress and anger in the treatment of phobias?

Over the course of several visits to discuss your phobia, a therapist will have the benefit of getting to know you well. Your primary care doctor may not be able to afford this luxury. Insights gained by a therapist can be communicated to your physician if you sign an authorization to allow such a discussion and ask that such communication take place. This team approach may lead to a more complete understanding of your condition and more successful treatment strategies.

A therapist typically wants to know everything about you: What was your upbringing like? How are your relationships working out? What is your educational level and how did you choose your career path? What problems run in your family? What kinds of trauma and stress have you faced in your life? What are all the physical symptoms you are experiencing? How do you perceive and interpret your feelings? What forms of treatment have you tried? Do you self-medicate?

It may take several sessions for a therapist to feel they understand what makes you tick. You will most likely be asked to fill out a number of questionnaires, and the therapist will probably perform a mental status evaluation (MSE). A basic MSE would include a description of your behavior and appearance, attitude toward the therapist, and details about your mood and emotional affect. Speech is evaluated for prosody, rate, and volume. You may be asked about perceptual disturbances and the therapist will be looking for any abnormality in thought process or content.

Level of alertness, orientation, memory, and other aspects of your sensorium and cognition are noted. Some comments will also be recorded on your impulse control, judgment, and reliability. Through this process of listening and learning, the therapist is trying to assess whether you have an emotional disorder, personality disorder, or any type of dysfunctional thought pattern. He or she is also developing an awareness of your strengths, resources, coping skills, and what support structure exists around you. Your therapist will formulate an assessment of your vulnerability and risk as well as your potential for recovery.

Be patient during these initial stages of therapy. You may know less about yourself than you think, and the process of getting to know you takes time and the benefit of professional training and insight. A counselor and therapist can then begin to give you feedback on your life situation, from marriage discord to how you feel about your career and other life choices. Ultimately, a counselor or therapist is most interested in how you feel about yourself. When the evaluation is complete, the therapist may recommend a variety of psychotherapeutic techniques.

COGNITIVE BEHAVIORAL THERAPY

Cognitive behavioral therapy (CBT) is the psychotherapeutic foundation of successful intervention for all types of phobias; stress and adjustment disorders; and many anxiety conditions, including post-traumatic stress disorder (PTSD), obsessive-compulsive disorder (OCD), panic disorder (PD), and generalized anxiety disorder (GAD). It has even been shown to benefit patients with chronic fatigue syndrome. The purpose of CBT is to resolve inhibitions, desensitize fears, and increase assertiveness. Ultimately, CBT allows the patient who has misconceptions and distorted thoughts and beliefs that fuel his or her anxiety to finally see the world accurately. Anxious patients commonly feel that they are the focus of scrutiny and attention, and that others are thinking critical thoughts about them. They often believe that their symptoms signal impending catastrophe and doom. These are the kinds of misconceptions that need CBT. Here is a brief explanation of how CBT helps specific problems:

Stress and Adjustment Disorders: CBT teaches stress-reduction techniques, and asks the patient to keep a daily log of stress precipitators. It teaches early recognition and removal from a source of stress before full-blown symptoms of anxiety occur. The technique of role-playing is sometimes used to help teach a new behavior response (such as assertiveness when asking for a raise), which needs to be practiced over and over again until it comes naturally.

Phobias: Systematic desensitization is a technique especially designed to decrease the patient's reactivity to a phobia. The therapist progressively exposes the patient to the phobic stimulus in a controlled environment to gradually reduce the anxiety experienced when in the presence of that stimulus. This is the emotional or experiential learning we were talking about at the beginning of this book. With agoraphobia and social phobia, it is especially important to counter the cognitive misperceptions of scrutiny and judgment by others.

GAD, PD, and OCD: With these anxiety disorders, the combination of medication with CBT is more effective than either alone. Behavioral techniques focus on altering the factors that precipitate an anxiety response and recognizing the secondary rewards that might support or encourage the patient's dysfunction. Desensitization by exposing the patient to graded doses of a phobic situation is effective and can be practiced by the patient at home. A study on OCD by University of California at Los Angeles researchers showed that CBT can actually change the way the brain functions and processes external stimuli. Twelve of 18 patients studied with OCD were found to have different brain scans after treatment compared to before treatment. The change was seen as significant to reduced activity in the caudate nucleus, an area of the brain known to be overactive in OCD.

Chronic Fatigue Syndrome (CBT): CBT was shown to help 70 percent of chronic fatigue patients improve their physical functioning and energy level in a study published in the March 1997 issue of the *American Journal of Psychiatry*. This means that much of the fatigue and physical impairments seen in chronic fatigue syndrome are really the result of anxious misperceptions and misinterpretations of what is going on inside the body. This waste of emotional energy contributes to the overall feeling of exhaustion and futility, and can be effectively countered by CBT.

COGNITIVE APPROACH TO THE TREATMENT OF PHOBIAS

Cognitive therapy focuses on patient misinterpretations, distorted perceptions and abnormal yet deeply held beliefs. Let's examine some examples of this kind of "wrong thinking." Replacing the untrue thought with the truthful reality is the focus of cognitive therapy:

Wrong thinking in the case of agoraphobia typically includes these presuppositions:

I have no control. Sooner or later we must accept the reality that many things are not under our control, nor should they be. "Control freaks" think they can lessen their anxiety by insisting on controlling every situation. This gives them difficulty in working and living with others. On the other hand, it is useful to recognize what we can and should control. While agoraphobics wish for a life that is spontaneous and free from fear, they focus on the opposite. They focus on the limitations imposed by the fear and their failure to control the fear, resulting in a life of self-confinement. The paradox is that the more energy you expend trying to control anxiety, the more fearful you will become.

I'm trapped. As with control, we must practice looking at how we are free instead of how we are trapped. Dismantling a false sense of entrapment begins with your perceptions. We are only trapped if we perceive that we have no options or choices. This is rarely the case, in reality. For example, of his many imprisonments, the Indian spiritual leader Mahatma Gandhi later stated that it was during these times that his mind and heart was most free to focus on the truth. Here, perception was the difference between four cold, stone walls and the limitless universe of the mind. Similarly, if you are temporarily confined in an airplane, train, or dentist's chair, it is probably wise to stay put and let your mind wander via a good book or visions of someplace you've always wanted to go. If you're in a movie theater, reassure yourself that if you had to leave, it would be no big deal. Others will not sense your anxiety or turn their focus to you (unless it is an exceptionally bad movie). In any case, people get up and leave a movie for a number of reasons, like to get a snack, go to the bathroom, call a friend, or just to stretch their legs. No one is inconvenienced or upset by this. Most people are subjected to the same constraints in a number of situations, but they don't feel anxious because they correctly perceive that there is no realistic danger, and therefore no need to escape.

My phobic anxiety will lead to a catastrophe. Fear of a catastrophe is the final component of agoraphobia. Whether it is death, complete humiliation, or insanity that will happen as a result of your anxiety symptoms, the fear of a catastrophe is your greatest fear and the strongest factor in the development of avoidance behaviors. In truth, most agoraphobics have experienced their anxiety symptoms many times, but have never experienced a catastrophe. Few can claim to have experienced death, insanity, or such humiliation that no one ever talked to them again. When it is said like this, the rational mind laughs and says. "Of course, it is unlikely a catastrophe will ever happen." But the emotional mind feels differently. It perceives itself as being unable to cope with what most of us would consider very "small catastrophes," such as being ridiculed for trembling or blushing during a wave of anxiety. CBT allows us to put our feared catastrophes back into perspective.

I am frail and vulnerable. You are what you think. In reality, it is just as easy to say, "I'm strong and a good survivor." Changing a negative into a positive thought is simply a matter of choice and repetition. All those times you told yourself you couldn't do it must now be replaced with the affirmative mindset over and over again. In truth, we all have inner strengths and abilities equal to the tasks we are asked to complete. In truth, we are all vulnerable to things that are beyond our control. There is no guarantee of security in this world, as the survivors of the December 26, 2004, tsunami will tell you. But they will also remind you that such risks are part of life and should not be used as an excuse for living a fearful, unfulfilled life. Tapping into our inner source of resourcefulness, strength, and power is the goal of therapy.

Typical wrong thinking in the case of specific phobias includes the following:

- "That plane/car/train/boat is unsafe. It could crash/sink/explode and that would be the end of me."

- "The injection will injure me or cause pain, and I might have an anxiety attack and faint."
- "The mice/spiders/cockroaches/birds may attack/bite/contaminate/kill me."

These thoughts are examples of irrational fears experienced by those with specific phobias. Even though they know the degree of fear and reaction is unreasonable given the level of the actual threat, these people cannot stop the response from happening. Although most of these fears must be unlearned by the experiential method, an attempt should be made to correct cognitive misperceptions about the real and true risk that the activity or object presents.

Wrong thinking in cases of social phobia includes these assertions:

I have no control in social situations. Social phobia patients often avoid social events because of a perceived inability to perform well in that environment. They realize that parties and social gatherings are not their strong suit, because they don't have the social skills to control that situation. They only see all the things that could go wrong, resulting in humiliation and embarrassment. Therapy tries to show social phobics the ways that they *do* have control. For instance, it would be natural to be fearful in a party with lots of new faces. Instead of saying, "There are too many people here that I don't know and I can't control all the judgment and scrutiny coming my way," say the real truth: "There are lots of people I don't know here, but I can go outside and distance myself if I need to. Actually, I can move around just fine, and it seems most people are not focused on me, but are just enjoying their conversations and having a good time. These people really aren't trying to bother me; they even seem friendly and polite." Remember that you can never control how others behave, only how you respond to their behavior. Assessing what you can and should control as opposed to what should be released and let go of is a focus of therapy.

I have to be perfect. Let's decide here and now that nobody is perfect, nor would they want to be. Not making mistakes means we are not challenging our potential. Being perfect is no fun either, and most people find perfection to be annoying and uncomfortable to be around. Accepting your faults allows you to laugh at yourself, which is a great way to endear yourself to others. Start having fun today by shedding your futile attempts at perfection.

Everyone is judging me. Get over it. People have better things to do with their time than think about you. Like you, most people are too busy scrutinizing themselves and dealing with their own problems to leave time for you and your problems. Remember the old 18–40–60 rule: When you're 18 years old, you hope nobody thinks negatively of you. When you're 40 years old, you don't give a damn about what anyone thinks about you. When you're 60 years old, you realize no one was ever thinking about you!

Anxiety and fear are weaknesses. Many carry the misperception that if they admit their phobias and fears, others will see them as emotionally weak. But bravery requires anxiety and fear to rise above and overcome. There is nothing more courageous than admitting and facing your fears. Inner strength and confidence comes from conquering these types of challenges. Dr. Gardner always felt uncomfortable speaking in front of others. "What if I say the wrong thing or give the wrong advice? They will all think I'm an idiot," he would tell himself. It was especially stressful, therefore, when he was asked to be a guest on a radio talk show with an estimated 1 million listeners. Finally deciding that he was as prepared as he could be, he let go of his anxiety and made the decision to enjoy the experience. He focused on the individuals calling in as though they were his friends or private patients, and ignored the thought of others listening in and judging. Because of this change in his thinking, he was able to relax and perform in a comfortable way that won him the position of a regular guest on the program. Dr. Gardner still remembers the surge of confidence that followed that first program, and how it has stayed with him to this day.

FOCUSING ON COGNITIVE BEHAVIORAL THERAPY FOR SOCIAL PHOBIA

Results of a voluminous amount of treatment–outcome data over the last ten years consistently supports the efficacy of two treatment modalities—cognitive behavioral therapy and pharmacotherapy—and suggests that they produce approximately equivalent outcomes (Gould et al. 1997). While we maintain that the combination of the two gives a faster and more complete result in the vast majority of patients, it is useful to review in more depth the modality of cognitive behavioral therapy (CBT) alone for social anxiety disorder (SAD). Much of what we learn in this section will also apply to the CBT approach to treating agoraphobia and specific phobia.

To avoid bogging down in repetition, we will focus only on the data for SAD, which is the most common type of phobia, and the phobia most likely to cause serious and often undiagnosed dysfunction. We have found that agoraphobia becomes such a problem that people seek help, while specific phobias often do not significantly impair functionality or quality of life to require treatment. Social phobia, however, can ruin lives if not diagnosed and treated. We feel social phobics are at high risk for avoiding therapy and resorting to substance abuse. Understanding how successful treatment has proven to be will hopefully change this.

Central to the cognitive behavioral model of social phobia are the self-perpetuating expectations of social failure, negative self-evaluations, increasing anxiety, and avoidance. Negative expectations about social situations often include fears that the anxiety will be uncontrollable (e.g., "I will be so nervous, I will faint, throw-up, or have to run off the stage"). In addition, the individual might believe that they will perform poorly (e.g., "I'm going to blow it again") and expect that others will evaluate them in a negative way (e.g., "People will think I'm stupid"). These patterns of anticipatory fears lead to increased anxious apprehension about social situations, which are the basis for avoidance behaviors.

Studies have shown that patients with SAD pay more attention to social–threat words and negative facial expressions. In short, they are focused on failure. They do not see the times they perform well socially, because they are busy anticipating a future failure or catastrophe. This overshadows any positive experience with the expectation of a negative experience, preventing a balanced picture of reality. For instance, a person with SAD may interpret their presentation as a disaster because they immediately picked up a grimace from a single member of the audience, while the approving nods and smiles of others escaped awareness altogether. We all make social mistakes, especially when we care too much about the outcome of a social interaction. We desperately want to make an impression on the little red-haired girl, or our boss or teacher. If we are too emotionally invested in the outcome, then success or failure matters greatly to us. This environment of emotional investment in the outcome, along with a history of negative experiences, is fertile ground for the anticipatory anxiety of the social phobic.

Those with SAD often have to work twice as hard as others to perform the task at hand and simultaneously maintain vigilance to feared potential outcomes. This is called the "dual task" mode. In addition, social phobics waste energy on increased self-focused attention and overestimate the degree to which their anxiety is perceptible to others (e.g., "they're all watching me squirm"). Minor failures, such as a quiver in the voice, are amplified and made the focus of attention, with negative interpretations of social failure being evoked (e.g., "Everyone heard my voice quiver and is thinking about how unprepared and nervous and stupid I am"). All of this energy and vigilance expended on negative thoughts makes it nearly impossible to stay on track with the social task at hand. We may then experience other failures, such as forgetting our train of thought. There is nothing more frightening to a presenter than drawing a complete blank. Social phobia patients will likely have certain "wrong thoughts," or cognitive misperceptions, that are responsible for amplifying small social events into social catastrophes. One scientist drew attention to three such "amplifying cognitions": 1) Even small errors mean that a person is defective, 2) being anxious in social situations is evidence that one is inept, and 3) any behavior that deviates from "normal" represents further evidence of dysfunction. These "amplifying beliefs" magnify existing concerns and cause additional anxiety (Otto 1999).

One of the natural consequences of this cycle of negative expectations and amplified anxiety is the urge to escape or avoid social situations. Avoidance behaviors and "safety strategies" prevent the social phobia patient from learning that negative outcomes do not occur. Instead of seeing that a social situation was successfully maneuvered, the social phobic perceives a narrow escape from an expected social catastrophe. Avoidance behaviors lock in the memories of social failure and prevent new learning that would disconfirm existing beliefs and negative expectations, The avoidance behaviors are learned to the exclusion of new social skills, causing further performance limitations. "Safety strategies" also appear to backfire. These behaviors include averting one's eyes while speaking (so as not to get overwhelmed by being looked at), speaking rapidly (so as not to freeze up in mid-sentence), or clenching one's hands (to hide trembling). One study demonstrated that these safety behaviors made the patient less likely to improve with exposure therapy (Wells et al. 1995). "Playing it safe" only teaches the social phobic that they can survive social situations with using lots of crutches, rather than learning that these behaviors are not needed to perform adequately.

CBT treatment of social phobia should 1) correct maladaptive or dysfunctional cognitions that produce anxious apprehension, 2) adjust core amplifying cognitions, 3) reduce attention to failure cues, 4) reduce

A cognitive-behavioral model of core patterns in social anxiety disorder

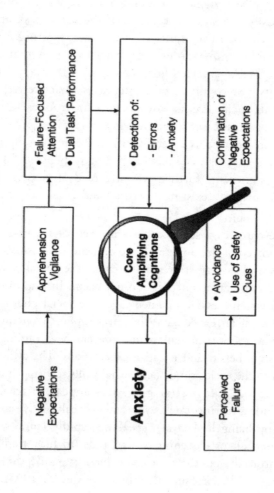

Figure adapted from Otto, M. W. (1999). Cognitive-behavioral therapy for social anxiety disorder: Model, methods, and outcome. Journal of Clinical Psychiatry, 60 (suppl. 9), 14-19.

avoidance and safety behaviors, and 5) increase exposure to, and accurate appraisal of, social performance and outcome. Treatment should also include social skills training and relaxation training.

CBT usually begins with informational intervention. During this stage of therapy, the patient is supplied with the cognitive behavioral model, emphasizing how dysfunctional thoughts lead to anxiety and avoidance behaviors. The second stage of therapy is cognitive restructuring, where the patient is asked to challenge the validity of their thoughts about themselves and the world based on real experience, rather that automatically accepting them as facts. Patients are shown how their thoughts can induce anxiety and lead to an unfavorable outcome. Patients are taught to identify self-defeating thoughts, such as those anticipating a negative performance ("I'm going to blow it"), those directed at a performance in progress ("I'm boring everyone, they think I'm an idiot"), and those ruminating over a past performance ("I sucked big time, as usual"). Once the patient has successfully identified these thought patterns, they can then stop the dysfunctional cognition and replacing it with a positive affirmation: "I'm going to do just fine." "People are appreciating my efforts and finding my presentation useful." "It wasn't perfect, but I'm improving." Patients also learn about cognitive distortions that are common in social phobia. One such distortion is that the way they feel about themselves is the way that they are perceived by others. For instance, the patient may feel they failed a social situation "because they felt anxious." In their view, experiencing anxiety is a negative outcome in itself, and an appropriate measure of social performance. Another distortion is the "all-or-nothing thinking," where the patient believes only two categories of outcomes are possible. In this mode of thinking, if a performance falls short of perfection, it means that they are a complete failure. The "mind reading" thought distortion involves the belief that one knows what others are thinking. Socially anxious patients often "just know" that others are judging them in a negative way, even in the absence of any objective evidence. The goal of cognitive restructuring is to get the patient to recognize and challenge their cognitive distortions—a brief period of silence during a conversation does not signal incompetence, and blushing in a social situation is not a catastrophe. Through accurate and logical thinking, the patient learns to appreciate that their social fears are unfounded, and that social situations need not be regarded as a threat.

Exposure Therapy: The Experiential/Emotional Learning Approach to the Treatment of Phobias

The efficacy of the previous cognitive interventions is supported in outcome studies; however, there is evidence that exposure interventions represent the most potent ingredient in CBT for social phobia (Feske and Chambless 1995; Gould et al. 1997; Taylor 1996).

Graded desensitization, or "exposure" therapy, is designed to help us unlearn the fear that our emotional mind has taught us. What we have learned through the emotional mind, we must unlearn through the emotional mind. Of course, this necessarily involves some degree of discomfort. Remember your first date? All the fuss and apprehension; the seeking of advice on what to do and when to do it; the heart pounding and palms sweating with anxiety and anticipation. We forced ourselves through this emotionally painful experience for what—so that we could convince ourselves or others that we were all grown-up? Because of some deep biological need overpowering our strong desire to call in sick? Whatever the reason, we did it, and we got through it. We worried about our manners, how we were chewing our food, the moments of uncomfortable silence, whether our hair was right, or if the spinach was stuck in our teeth. And in the end, we worried if we would we get that first real kiss or a peck on the cheek. Most of us got the kiss and were willing to try again. And each time we got a little better at it. It got less and less uncomfortable and more fun. Self-esteem grew as we began to like ourselves better.

This is an example of how emotional learning through fear and discomfort ultimately can lead to new skills and confidence. And that's what life is all about: growth. Exposure therapy is like that first date: we want to grow, but we wish we could skip that awkward and anxious process. But that's how we are programmed to learn. Growth takes courage and the acceptance of the risk of emotional pain. Only with experiential learning are we effectively engaging our entire being in the process of learning and growth.

Exposure intervention guides the patient as they systematically confront the feared situation. In the case of social phobia, the patient is helped through the process of entering the social situation, allowing the fear to dissipate naturally by remaining in the situation, and then interpreting the fear accurately and performing adequately. By not prematurely escaping from or avoiding the social situation, the patient learns a sense of safety and increased confidence. Cognitive insights should have already been absorbed so that negative thoughts that arise during the exposure can be effectively challenged.

Exposure therapy is highly personalized and proceeds to increasingly difficult tasks. The exposure task is rehearsed in a role-playing session, and dysfunctional thoughts and expectations are identified and reviewed by the therapist. Alternative cognitive responses that are more positive and adaptive are generated and practiced. When the patient feels comfortable with the initial, limited exposure situations, he or she progresses to more difficult and challenging tasks. The patient is also instructed to shift their attention away from themselves (what they are thinking or feeling about the situation) to what is actually occurring (i.e., listening to others and watching their behavior).

In addition, therapy is directed at assessing the patients' beliefs about the likelihood of their feared catastrophes, identifying the avoidance and safety behaviors, showing that expected negative outcomes do not occur, gradually eliminating safety behaviors during exposure exercises, and reviewing the exposure as to what was learned (e.g., the catastrophe did not happen). In addition, the therapist and patient should agree on the behavioral goals for the exposure exercise. For example, in a simulated exposure to meeting a stranger at a small party, the behavioral goals may be (a) to say hello and introduce yourself, (b) to maintain good eye contact, and (c) to successfully break off the conversation and continue mingling. Even though they may feel anxiety, the patient is usually able to accomplish the preset goals. This reinforces the notion that feelings of anxiety are not appropriate measures of social performance. You can still have a successful and positive social experience while feeling nervous and insecure. Successful exposures allow positive memories to build as expectations are revised and corrected, providing the foundation for increased confidence in future social interactions.

THE USE OF VIRTUAL REALITY IN EXPOSURE THERAPY

Intuitively, you might think that virtual reality exposure therapy would be ineffective. After all, how can you fool your brain into thinking that that computer-generated images inside a helmet is real. Well, apparently it's not about fooling your rational, prefrontal cortex. The amygdala and hippocampus seem to respond to virtual reality exposure much like real-life exposure to a feared situation, showing gradual unlearning and extinction of the phobic fear response after multiple sessions. Virtually Better is a virtual reality laboratory and treatment center in Decatur, Georgia. Here, phobic clients are able to speak in front of a large audience, sit in a crowded airplane, cross a primitive wooden bridge high above a raging river, or walk through a room full of spiders—all while never leaving the comfort of their office chair. The days when a therapist needed to accompany the client while driving through the tunnel, crossing the bridge, or riding in the elevator may be coming to an end. Virtual reality therapy, because it is cost-effective and readily accessible, is quickly becoming mainstream for the treatment of specific and social phobias.

THE TEACHING OF SOCIAL SKILLS

Most people with social phobia do not lack social skills; they just don't always apply them due to the distraction of anxiety or the presence of avoidance behaviors. The teaching of social skills, therefore, is really meant for those who demonstrate a clear deficit. The teaching of social skills first incorporates education about social interactions and the behaviors required to achieve positive results. The patient then rehearses these behaviors in role-playing sessions with the therapist. For example, the role-play may be to rehearse how to properly introduce oneself in a social situation. After the role-play, the therapist will offer corrective feedback about the patient's performance. Problems including maintaining eye contact, speaking in an audible voice, and observing social conventions such as shaking hands would be addressed at this time. Social skills training sessions are, by their very nature, exposure experiences, where the patient benefits from learning in a trusted and controlled environment.

FAMILY AND GROUP THERAPY

In Heimberg's group treatment program (Heimberg et al. 1990; 1995), exposure therapy was conducted in the context of a group setting, during weekly 2.5-hour sessions. This provided a ready-made learning experience, using other group members for constructing simulation exercises. For instance, some group members could role-play the audience while others gave short speeches. Other times they might set up a special situation relevant to a particular member's phobia, such as the attending of a formal dinner party. There is a sense of safety and support in being in a group in which all are facing the same affliction, and therefore cannot be judgmental. Many actresses, actors, and performance artists remember putting on shows for their families when they were kids. Of course, the captive audience smiled and clapped with wild enthusiasm, causing a surge of self-confidence. Not all of us had this supportive family experience, and must now get it through group therapy.

In our clinic, we have found family therapy especially helpful. First off, we have a group that already has been introduced (without the stigmatizing "Hi, my name is Brian and I have a phobia..."). Secondly, we can evaluate the interpersonal family dynamic that our patient lives with every day. Teaching the entire family about the nature of phobias and the rationale of our treatment strategy is a way to get everyone on the same page. There is no benefit in pushing someone into an uncomfortable exposure without preparation, as some family members may want to do. There is no place for unkind or disparaging remarks, or even for playful teasing. Instead, getting the family to work as a team pulling on the same end of the rope is the goal of family therapy. Teaching each member how they can reinforce the proper cognitions and help the patient challenge their misperceptions is especially helpful. Using the family as a "safe" audience for the patient to practice on is an added plus. Giving the patient a home environment that is kind and supportive is priceless.

COUNSELING FOR STRESS AND ANGER MANAGEMENT

As we have learned, the inability to cope successfully with stress and anger damages our emotional nervous system as well as cardiovascular system and makes life difficult for everyone around us. So where's the pay-off? Why do we allow ourselves to get worked-up, stressed-out, and upset over things that really don't matter? Regarding stress, much of the pressures and frustrations that we perceive are completely self-imposed. We take responsibility for everything and everybody. Anything that goes wrong is our fault. We insist on an unrealistic level of performance and perfection. Our priorities are all wrong, as we often lose track of what really has meaning and chase after manufactured measures of success. The anxiety that follows may be nature's (or God's) way of telling you to look inside at your belief system and reassess your choices and direction in life. A therapist may ask you, "What will really be remembered and matter 20 years from now?" A good therapist will help you get back to your core values and beliefs. From here, you can begin putting life back into a healthy balance. Another cause of undue stress is our failure to seek help and advice. We wait until we are overwhelmed and at our wit's end, or have lost our job or marriage before getting the support we need. Stress management teaches us to recognize the signs of overload before we become dysfunctional and experience irrevocable loss. Recognizing our limitations, setting up boundaries, setting reasonable goals and expectations, learning organizational skills, and identifying our resources and support structures are all helpful elements of stress-management counseling. Teaching the relaxation response through hypnotherapy, biofeedback, meditation, and deep-breathing exercises can enhance the benefits of stress-management therapy.

Anger is often a dysfunctional means of coping with or attempting to control our environment. Unfortunately, it usually backfires on us, leading to social isolation, rejection, personal failures, and less control over our lives. The basic notion of karma seems to hold valuable truth for living. The match that touches off explosions of anger can be any of the following: 1) an unrealistic expectation of the way things should be, and 2) an inflated sense of self-importance. For instance, a person with road rage has the unrealistic expectation that everyone should respect their time schedule and get out of the way, and the firm conviction that where they are going and what they are doing is more important than anyone else's plans. This erroneous way of thinking causes us to trigger our anger centers whenever the world does not conform to our expectations, or we feel others don't recognize our importance.

The "three Rs" for managing anger are:

1. *Reframing* expectations and deciding what is really important to get angry about and what is not (choose your battles wisely).

2. *Relaxing* physically and taking a deep breath and pausing before reacting emotionally with anger.

3. *Responding rationally* and using the higher brain (cortex) to inform the emotions what the appropriate reaction to the situation should be. (The higher frontal cortex area takes over 20 years to complete development, which makes responding rationally difficult for children and adolescents.)

Chapter 9

USING THE ANXIETY TOOLBOX TO CONQUER PHOBIAS

This chapter answers four questions:

1. What dietary habits can help in the treatment of phobias?
2. What vitamins and supplements are sometimes used in the treatment of phobias?
3. How can you achieve a positive mindset to combat phobias?
4. What are other accessible, easy-to-use tools to fight back against phobias?

Pernicious phobias can be extinguished simply by our choice of lifestyle—a choice we all make among several options available to us. Losing our vulnerability to anxiety and phobias directly depends on our ability to make the correct choices in our relationships, careers, financial dealings, parenting responsibilities, and in our diet, exercise, and health matters. Every choice we make should be informed by the answer to a simple question: *Which response will best serve my emotional health?* If faced with a bottle of scotch while feeling anxious or depressed, the decision that best serves emotional health is to just say no.

Being mindful about our choices at each moment and consistently opting for the positive, health-affirming direction is a chore at first. Later, after much practice, the right choices will come without effort because we are thinking from a well and balanced mind that recognizes the benefit of making the right lifestyle decisions.

In the process of making such lifestyle choices, we will frequently confront the issue of stress. Here there is bad news and good news. The bad news: we create our own stress. The good news: we create our own stress.

PHOBIA-KILLING DIET

A well-balanced, nontoxic diet is essential for reducing the stress and anxiety that fuels our phobias. First we must eliminate an overreliance on stimulants in the diet so that our nervous system has a chance to calm down. Here are the main culprits:

Caffeine: Found in many products, such as coffee, chocolate, tea, and soda, caffeine causes the release of adrenalin, which in turn increases anxiety and tension. Gradually reduce and eliminate caffeine from your diet. Abrupt discontinuation can cause withdrawal symptoms such as headaches, nausea, and tremors.

Alcohol: Alcohol is one of the most common forms of "self-medication" for phobias. Alcohol also stimulates the release of adrenalin, as well as insulin. The short-term effects of sedation are soon replaced by nervous tension, irritability, mood swings, and insomnia. Excess alcohol will increase the fat deposits in the heart and liver, and suppresses the activity of the immune system. Because of its effects of liver metabolism, alcohol allows stress hormones produced by the adrenal glands to circulate longer in the bloodstream, increasing the level of damage to the nervous and cardiovascular systems.

Sugar: Sugar is the simplest of the "simple carbohydrates," so named because their simple structure allows quick absorption and metabolism. Sugars are often used as a quick energy or mood booster, but research shows there is a heavy price to be paid. As the most potent stimulator of pancreatic insulin production, sugar creates a situation of sugar overload followed an hour or two later by a sudden drop in the blood sugar level. These insulin and sugar roller-coasters are responsible for the release of stress hormones from the adrenal glands. They are also responsible for an unhealthy balance of prostaglandin proteins that contribute to lowered immune resistance, as well as negative mood and anxiety states.

Fat: Fat is a calorie-dense food that lowers the metabolism and is a primary player in the development of obesity and cardiovascular disease. Too much fat gets deposited in the liver, where it interferes with the cleansing and metabolic activities of that organ. Fat is believed to increase the likelihood of developing a variety of malignancies, including cancer of the colon, breast, and prostate.

Complex Carbohydrates: Increasing complex carbohydrates will help stabilize blood sugar levels and will trigger brain serotonin release, promoting a sense of relaxation. Complex carbohydrates include brown rice, wild rice (actually not a true rice grain), and whole grains (oats, wheat, etc.). Simple carbohydrates should be reduced or avoided because they cause increased fluctuations of blood sugar levels, contribute to weight gain, and are responsible for triggering anxiety states. These foods include sugar itself, as well as anything made from processed flour (bread, pasta, pastries, baked goods), and fruit juice.

Fruits and Vegetables: Fresh fruit, rather than fruit juice, especially if vine-ripened, contains important antioxidant phytochemicals. Enjoy two to three seasonal fresh fruits per day. Green, yellow, and orange vegetables are all rich in minerals, vitamins, and phytochemicals, which boost the immune response and help protect against disease. Vegetables also enhance the absorption of the amino acid L-tryptophan, the precursor of serotonin, thereby increasing serotonin production.

Diet Summary

Foods to Eat: Eat complex carbohydrates such as whole grains, limited fresh fruits, and plenty of vegetables. Legumes (beans) are good sources of protein. Soybeans can be found in a wide variety of products, including miso soup, tofu, and soy milk. Lean dairy and meats are also good sources of protein, and protein helps to stabilize blood sugar levels. Too much animal protein can elevate levels of the norepinephrine and dopamine neurotransmitters in the brain, which can cause higher levels of anxiety in some individuals.

Foods to Avoid: Avoid coffee and other caffeinated beverages. Black tea has less than one-third of the caffeine and none of the harmful oils. For those who are currently addicted to coffee, this is a good choice. Fried foods and foods rich in fat are immune suppressing and contribute to obesity and fatigue. Sugar and other simple carbohydrates contribute to anxiety by causing wide fluctuations in blood sugar levels. Alcohol triggers adrenal release of stress hormones, interferes with healthy sleep cycles, slows liver filtering processes, and lowers immune system response. By all these mechanisms, it can increase anxiety and stress in vulnerable individuals. That is why you should never drink when depressed or anxious, or as a treatment for stress.

Vitamins and Supplements

Although health store or supermarket vitamins and supplements are hardly ever the cure-all they are held to be by some enthusiasts, these chemicals, such as prescribed drugs, can exert an influence on physical and mental health. Discuss any regimen of vitamins or supplements with your doctor. A brief list of vitamins and supplements for phobias and related conditions follows:

For Anxiety, Irritability, and Insomnia: Niacin (vitamin B-3), vitamin B-6, vitamin B-15, folic acid, choline, L-tryptophan, vitamin A, bet carotene, chromium, inositol, B-complex, calcium and magnesium, silicon, multiple vitamin/mineral supplement, and manganese.

For Depression and Fatigue: Vitamin B-12 (preferably given by injection), B-complex, calcium, calcium and magnesium, flower essence, pyridoxine (B-6), thiamine (B-1), niacin (B-3), choline, chromium, vanadium, zinc, lecithin, iodine, potassium, essential fatty acids, vitamin C, L-tyrosine, folic acid, and inositol.

For Stress: B-complex (especially B-2, B-5, B-6, and B-15), folic acid, vitamin C with bioflavonoids, vitamin E, calcium, magnesium, lecithin, phosphorus, Bach flower remedy, zinc potassium, and L-tyrosine.

For Bipolar Disorder: amino acids such as L-tyrosine and L-taurine, B-complex, mineral complex, iodine, chromium, vanadium, B-2, B-6, B-12, vitamin C with bioflavonoids, calcium and magnesium, potassium, and essential fatty acids.

Choosing a Positive Mindset

Avoid negative thoughts of powerlessness, dejection, failure, and despair. Chronic stress makes us vulnerable to negative suggestion. Learn to focus on the positives. Here are a few tips:

Focus on Your Strengths. We all have particular training, gifts, talents, and background experience that we bring into a particular dilemma. Sometimes we get away from our positive resources, which is like fighting a battle without our best troops. Think about where you stand. What real estate is beneath your feet that you own? Once you know this, utilize it to get where you want to go.

Learn From the Stress You Are Under. Stress and anxiety are our greatest teachers because they teach our emotional brain through experiential learning—the most efficient and powerful learning of all. Every stressful situation has a lesson to teach us, if we are willing to learn. If we fail to recognize and learn these lessons, we are doomed to repeat our mistakes. Think about which decisions or actions led to the stress you are under. What might you do differently in the future to avoid this?

Look for Opportunities in Stressful Situations. Sometimes insight comes when we are in the midst of stress, a thought or idea we may never have recognized if we were not sensitized by the experience of anxiety. Be open to the learning process at all times.

Choose to Be Positive. Seek out the positive. Embrace the positive. First decide if you have the ability to change the stressful situation. If you do, then go ahead and have the courage to make a change. You have control. Procrastination is the root cause of many stressful situations. If you have no control on the outcome, don't worry about it. Let the situation resolve itself—there's nothing you can do anyway. This thought is reflected by the "Serenity Prayer" of the theologian Rheinhold Niebuhr, adopted by Alcoholics Anonymous:

> God, grant me the serenity to accept the things I cannot change:
> The courage to change the things I can;
> And the wisdom to know the difference—
> Living one day at a time;
> Accepting hardships as the pathway to peace.

Remember that stress and negativity are choices you make. Every day we choose to be happy, sad, angry, irritable, relaxed, and so forth. Choosing to look at the positive side of life will save us a great deal of wasted emotional energy on things of the past that we have no ability to change. In the words of Ram Dass, "Be here now." And keep on practicing being positive. Pythagoras said, "Choose always the way that seems the best, however rough it may be. Custom will soon render it easy and agreeable."

Learn to Forgive and Move On. Forgiving yourself and others is a necessary tool in living a successful, happy life. Don't hold grudges; they only poison your life.

Learn to live in the present.

REFRAMING

Reframing is a technique used to change the way we look at things in order to feel better about them. The key to reframing is to recognize that there are many ways to interpret the same situation ("The glass is half full or half empty"). Focusing on the positive, eliminating the negative, and latching onto the affirmative by enjoying each moment is a gift that some people are born with and others need to practice mindfully on a daily basis. Reframing our problems in the context of our spiritual beliefs can be a great coping strategy for those who choose a religious context for their living. For instance, if you believe that everything happens for a reason and is the will of God, you can give your burdens over to God to help you sort them out. You don't have to activate your stress response and flood your bloodstream with stress hormones.

BEING ASSERTIVE

Nonassertiveness allows others to walk all over you, leaving you frustrated and emotionally bruised. You are surrendering control of the situation to others, who probably are not looking out for your best interests. Being assertive means standing up for your personal rights and expressing your thoughts, feelings, and beliefs directly, honestly, and spontaneously in ways that don't infringe on the rights of others. Assertive people respect themselves and others. They take responsibility for their actions and choices. In the face of failure, they are disappointed, but retain their sense of self-confidence and self-worth. Assertive people are able to recognize when others are trying to use or manipulate them, and are able to politely decline to become involved. Assertive people recognize when it is appropriate to help others, and when it is reasonable for others to take responsibility for their own problems. Assertiveness training is widely available and proves to be a useful tool for any anxiety toolbox.

SAYING NO TO DESTRUCTIVE RELATIONSHIPS

Part of being assertive means choosing relationships that are healthy, meaningful, and uplifting, while just saying *no* to destructive, disrespectful, "needy," or downright selfish partners.

GETTING ORGANIZED AND
MANAGING TIME SUCCESSFULLY

One of the most common causes of stress is being disorganized at work or at home. Here are some tips on how to get organized:

Keep a Diary. Try to articulate your personal and career goals. Express your values and priorities. What do you want out of life, and what options do you see in accomplishing your goals.

Write Lists of Tasks to Accomplish. Prioritize them and schedule dates for completion based on which tasks will reduce stress most (e.g., finding a job would come before cleaning the garage). Separate the list into long-term vs. short-term tasks. The short-term list should be just the things you want to complete today, and should not have more than five items.

Learn to Have Fewer Needs and Wants. The more you think you need and want, the less satisfied and more anxious you will become. Look at all your bills to see what products and services you really need and which you could learn to live without, at least until you are well organized and financially secure. In a relationship, both partners must agree to curb their spending and work together on the goal of simplifying and stabilizing their life together. Practicing a little self-denial can be a confidence-builder, and if you can keep it up for about five years, you'll be able to enjoy those things you denied yourself without guilt or worry about how you will be able to afford them.

Get Rid of Clutter. One of Suze Orman's best-selling books, *The Courage to be Rich*, focuses on her simple rule of cleaning the clutter out of your life. In her opinion, money cannot flow into your life until you have cleaned away the obstacles that crowd in around you. Hold a few garage sales. Get rid of every piece of clothing, appliance, toy, book, and box of papers that you really have no need for in the future. Get rid of junk that clutters your rooms and hallways and storage closets. The art of feng shui is often used in architectural design to make sure that a space allows the flow of positive energy and thoughts. Clutter creates a serious blockage to our ability to think clearly and feel emotional peace.

Learn to Say No. Your job is to clean up the old clutter and organize and simplify your existence, *not* to take on new projects, obligations, or responsibilities. Until you have career, financial, family, and health goals on target, you have no business extending yourself further. You won't be able to help anyone else until you have your life in ship-shape. Learn to draw the line and be assertive. Get help when you can and delegate tasks to others when appropriate. Have your husband make his own sandwich and ask your daughter if she can find another ride home from volleyball practice. Realize you can't keep doing everything for everybody. Explain to your boss that you would like to take on more, but you have other obligations to fulfill first. Explain to your boss you can take on a new task only if you are able to give up another task, and give him the choice as to which he would prefer you to do.

Pad Your Schedule. Realize that everything takes more time than you anticipated. Allotting extra time to complete a task, arrive at the airport, get to work, or meet a deadline will reduce anxiety and stress significantly.

Decide When to Turn Off Perfectionism. Sometimes perfectionism is necessary, especially when we are emotionally invested in the product or outcome. The old saying "if you want it done right, do it yourself" applies here. Whether painting a landscape, making a gourmet dinner, writing a speech, or performing surgery, a level of perfectionism is required. Other times, perfectionism gets in the way of efficiency and blocks our view of the big picture of what we need to accomplish. You don't have to do everything with meticulous detail, and insisting to do so is a sign of inflexibility that leads to unnecessary stress.

Take Breaks. Giving yourself short physical and mental breaks throughout the day that take you away from the stress of work or home responsibilities will make you more focused and productive.

Don't Make Big Decisions When You Are Stressed. Major decisions that might change your life should not be made when you are overtired, anxious, or depressed. Instead, focus your energy on smaller tasks and lesser decisions that are aimed at getting stress under control and improving your emotional and physical health.

LIVING WITHIN YOUR BUDGET

Financial responsibility is an admired trait in an individual, and an illusive goal and promise of many politicians. Living within your budget shows a level of maturity and humility that is quickly rewarded by the laws of nature. Within a short time, we feel the liberating relief of not owing anybody anything. Much of our anxiety is directly related to our financial health. Showing respect for our money is the same as showing respect for ourselves. Wasting or spending money we don't have shows that we are not in touch with the reality of who we are, and anxiety and stress will be the price we pay. Until we learn the lesson of financial responsibility, we are doomed to a life of worrying about never having enough, of living in fear of the future.

REGULAR EXERCISE

Research has shown that physical exercise is a powerful stress reliever. There is nothing quite as helpful as exercise is easing stress and preparing the mind and body for the trials of everyday life. Exercise strengthens the heart, lowers the blood pressure, increases the elasticity of the blood vessels, improves oxygen supply to the tissues, and also lowers the blood level of harmful lipids that cause hardening of the arteries. Mentally, exercise provides a release of negative emotions such as anger, frustration, and irritability, leading to a more balanced and positive outlook. The positive effects of exercise on our emotions can be directly attributed by the chemical changes in the brain and body caused by exercise. While reducing the amount of adrenal stress hormones circulating in the bloodstream, exercise triggers greater release of endorphins, the powerful, pain-relieving, mood-elevating chemicals in the brain. Exercise keeps the body functioning properly and promotes deep and restful sleep.

Exercise has another benefit: it stops you from worrying. Exercise gives the emotional areas of the brain involved in stress and worry a chance to rest and renew so that they are able to perform when needed in the future. There are many other ways to "rest your mind," including dancing, listening to music, reading, working on a craft or hobby, playing a musical instrument, meditating, and getting a massage. It could be argued that man invented all of these activities with the primary purpose and goal of relieving stress and tension by distracting the mind from its worries.

Like anything else, exercise can be overdone. A person who is in the gym every day or who needs to do extreme levels of physical activity is probably battling a stress disorder. For those who are mostly sedentary, increasing exercise has many health benefits. For those who are already physically exhausted from overworking or a physically demanding job, additional exercise makes no sense. In designing your exercise program, consider the following advice:

Choose an Exercise You Enjoy. Mountain biking, swimming, hiking, speed walking, and kayaking are all good choices. You must find an activity that you can perform consistently and that is fun. If it is the right program, you will miss it and look forward to your next session if you skip a day.

Choose Activities That Bring You Into Contact With Other People. The gym or special interest clubs are excellent ways to get connected to others and the community.

Do Some Aerobic Exercise For Ten to 30 Minutes Three, to Five Times a Week. Aerobic exercise is sustained activity involving the major muscle groups, such as swimming, running, or brisk walking. Additional aerobic activities include sports such as tennis, volleyball, soccer, yoga, t'ai chi, and some forms of martial arts. This kind of exercise strengthens your cardiovascular system and increases overall strength and stamina. The goal of aerobic exercise is for your pulse to reach a training rate that is appropriate for your age. Start out with five minutes, three times a week, and try to gradually work up to a 20- to 30-minute session.

Do Some Anaerobic Exercises Two to Six Days a Week. There are three types of anaerobic exercise. Isotonic exercise occurs when your muscles contract against a resistance with movement, as in weight lifting. Weight lifting causes tiny tears in the muscle being exercised that take several days to rebuild and strengthen. This process builds increased muscle mass and causes our body metabolism to increase, thereby burning off fat, even on the days we are not lifting. Isometrics involves contracting your muscles against a resistance without movement. Isometrics increases muscle strength and tone without increasing muscle bulk. Calisthenics are stretching exercises, like sit-ups, toe-touches, and knee-bends. These exercises help increase flexibility and joint mobility. All forms of aerobic and anaerobic exercise reduce stress effectively. The kind of exercises you choose depends on your personal preferences and your physical ability. Isotonic exercises should be limited to two times a week, as the body needs time to recover. Isometrics and calisthenics can be done every day, if time allows. Always get a complete physical exam from your physician before embarking on a new or vigorous exercise program.

YOGA

Yoga is best known as a set of physical practices that include gentle stretches, breathing practices, and progressive relaxation. These physical practices are intended to ready the body and mind for meditation, as well as help you develop a meditative perspective on life. These meditative practices also follow a sequence. First developed is the capacity to withdraw the senses from focus on the outer world, then the capacity to concentrate on a meditative subject—a candle flame, a sacred or uplifting word or image, or the movement of the breath. Finally, and for most of us only occasionally, the concentration leads into a wordless and timeless experience of inner peace. The yoga masters describe various subtleties among these states of inner peace, but most of us, at best, achieve moments of this experience only from time to time.

Before participating in the mind–body therapy known as yoga, one should have some knowledge of the underlying philosophy of this practice. The yogis believe that we are all searching for happiness, but that most of us settle for the watered-down version of brief and transient pleasures. The yogis believe that in some stage of our spiritual evolution over many lifetimes we will become dissatisfied with these temporary pleasures and begin a quest for eternal bliss. Methods to achieve this were developed and perfected by the yogis thousands of years ago. They consider that the laws of nature are so designed that we have no choice but to evolve. In the early stages, nature uses pain as the main mechanism for this spiritual evolution. Eventually, we find that the things of the world—money, sex, relationships, drugs and alcohol, or fame, for example—do not produce happiness or a sense of purpose, and we will start looking more deeply into life for answers. In the later stages of spiritual evolution, we no longer need pain to spur us on. Each stage of progress produces such an enhanced sense of peace and happiness that we look forward to the next level. Instead of pain, reward becomes the prime motivator. Yoga philosophy is so comprehensive that it deals with every aspect of life and delves into the very nature of reality.

In practice, yoga is an applied science of the mind and body. It comes from the Hindu Vedas (scriptures). Practice and study of it helps to bring about a natural balance of body and mind so that a healthy state can manifest itself. Yoga itself does not create health; rather, it creates an internal environment that allows the individual to come to his own state of dynamic balance, or health. Basically, yoga teaches that a healthy person is a harmoniously integrated unit of body, mind, and spirit. Therefore, good health requires a simple, natural diet, exercise in fresh air, a serene and untroubled mind, and an awareness that man's deepest and highest self is an image of the spirit of God. For some, yoga becomes a philosophy that offers instruction and insight, but for others, yoga is equally satisfying as a physical therapy alone.

For our purposes, one of the most beneficial applications of yoga is in relieving stress and fatigue, and its use in relaxation therapy. Indra Devi, author of many books on yoga, suggests that with yoga "you will be able to enjoy better sleep, a happier disposition, a clearer and calmer mind. You will learn how to build up your health and protect yourself against colds, fevers, constipation, headaches, fatigue, and other troubles. You will know what to do in order to remain youthful, vital and alert, regardless of your calendar age...." The clinical benefits have been well documented in a myriad of respected studies on such divergent problems as asthma, premenstrual tension, heart disease, obesity, diabetes, alcoholism, tobacco addiction, stomach ulcers, high blood pressure, back pain, arthritis, and the development of cancer. In addition, yoga has been found to improve cognitive mental performance and reduce subjective complaints of fatigue, depression, anxiety, and stress. Yoga can be a ready and enjoyable tool to combat any number of physical or emotional ailments. Whether to help keep on track with a diet, quit smoking, improve concentration while studying or taking an exam, or melt away stressful emotions, yoga is an ancient, tried and true remedy.

In our study of phobias, we are especially interested in the effects of yoga on the experience of fear. Most of us succumb at some point to fears and anxieties. We are more vulnerable to these emotions if we are run down by stress in the form of physical and mental exhaustion. The goal of yoga is fearless, confident living. Its aim is to replace worry and pessimism with a "yea-saying" appreciation of life and acceptance of the universe. Fear is replaced by the positive mental values of poise, contentedness, patience, assurance, and faith in life. By recurrent, regular efforts to reduce tension through yoga exercises, we may stay and finally reverse our tendency toward emotional illness derived from unrelenting fear. The long-range goal of yoga is not just momentary relaxation, but the living of a relaxed life; not merely momentary mental agility, but an agile life; not just momentary pliability, but a continuingly pliable existence; not just momentary relief from disturbance, but a permanently peaceful perspective.

Spiritual perspective has long been recognized as a useful tool in reducing vulnerability to stress, anxiety, and depression. Yoga may help develop a stronger spiritual framework to fall back on at times of stress and disappointment, no matter what your individual religious beliefs might be. In *Christian Yoga*, Dechanet, a Roman Catholic monk who was led into yoga by his Catholic predecessors, gives a vivid account of how he uses yogic techniques as aids to worship. He describes "a euphoria that pervades the story of my experiment. I wish to make it clear that this euphoria is real and lasting and spreads through the various levels of my daily life, physical, psychical, and spiritual" (HarperCollins, 2000). Even though few of us will achieve anything like perpetual exuberance, ecstatic joy, or euphoria, attainment of a more trustful, positive outlook on life provides a more fertile soil for spiritual growth.

MEDITATION

Most of the people who learn meditation do so because of the beneficial effects on stress. Stress hormones have been shown to decrease during meditation, and remain stabilized for some time afterward. This translates directly into a reduction of anxiety and a nervous system that is not as vulnerable to the fear response that is triggered by phobias. Other psychological benefits attributed to meditation include decreased depression, irritability, and moodiness; improved learning and memory; increased self-actualization; increased energy and sense of vitality; increased happiness; and overall emotional stability.

By simple definition, meditation is engagement in contemplation, especially of a spiritual or devotional nature. The mind is trained to focus inward on a single form or idea, to the exclusion of all other forms, thoughts, and ideas. The aspirant attempts to minimize perceptions through the senses (i.e., touch, sight, and hearing). The goal of meditation is to quiet the mind and disconnect it from the constant barrage of external and internal stimulation. In studies on yoga, Zen Buddhism, and transcendental meditation (TM), scientists have come to the conclusion that meditation is a "wakeful, hypo-metabolic state." They found that:

1. Yogis could slow both heart rate and the rate of perspiration.
2. Yogis could slow the rate of metabolism as confirmed by decreased oxygen consumption and carbon dioxide output.
3. Electroencephalogram (EEG) recordings of the brain waves of meditating yogis showed an increase in the calm "alpha rhythm" waves during both eyes closed and eyes open recordings.
4. The skin resistance to electrical stimulation was increased (indicating increased tolerance to external stimuli).

Recall for a moment our natural fight or flight mechanism of dealing with stressful situations. Our brain neurochemicals of norepinephrine and dopamine are activated, as well as our adrenal gland output of adrenalin and cortisol, due to the activation of the sympathetic nervous system. This activation causes a decrease in brain alpha waves and an increase in the stimulating beta waves as the brain prepares to flee on foot or stand and fight. In our modern lives, such a fearful or violent reaction is rarely helpful or necessary. These instinctive defense–alarm reactions often do not serve our cause well, and would be best replaced by more calm and serene reactions of equanimity and fearlessness. Such desirable reactions of nonaggression and peaceful attitude are generated by yoga and meditation.

PRACTICING GRATITUDE

Expressing gratitude is a form of embracing the positive, and always seeing the glass as "half full." Don't forget to practice gratitude for all the good things in your life. While you are enjoying a life experience, such as good food and drink, a cold glass of water, a restful nap, the feeling of fresh air filling your lungs, the view of a beautiful sunset, or the sound of the cheerful voice of someone you love, remember that all this can and will be taken away from you someday. Imagine what it would be like to be deprived of these things and how much you would miss them. Then let yourself feel a sense of gratitude that you were able to have that experience. Gratitude goes a long way in putting our minds and hearts in the proper perspective to view our life situations and keep negative impulses such as self-pity, irritability, unkindness, and arrogance in check.

HEALTHY SLEEP HYGIENE

Basic guidelines for overcoming insomnia and achieving restful, healthy sleep include the following:

1. Keep a regular schedule of when you go to bed and when you get up.
2. Avoid afternoon naps that keep you from falling asleep at night.
3. Do your exercise in the morning, not late in the day.
4. Avoid alcohol and caffeine within six hours of bedtime.
5. Use the bedroom for sleep and sex. Don't read, watch TV, do paperwork, answer the phone, have arguments, or do anything stressful in the sleep environment.
6. Make sure the bedroom is quiet and comfortable. If you live in a noisy area, buy a device to create "white noise," such as a fan.
7. Go to bed in a relaxed mood. If you're not relaxed, consider eating a snack high in carbohydrates, such as grains, legumes, pasta, bread, vegetables, fruits, or a bowl of cereal.

8. Don't lie in bed awake, thinking and worrying. Get up and leave the bedroom, go to the bathroom, eat a snack, or watch part of the late-night movie. When you feel sleepy and relaxed, go back to the bedroom.

STICKING TO A REGIMEN WITH RHYTHM

Don't forget that our bodily functions and brain chemistry is under the influence of our circadian rhythms directed by the chemical and neurological output of our pineal glands. This means we are designed to be on a cycle and that we will perform better emotionally and physically if we adhere to our natural rhythms. An easy way to do this is make sure you go to bed and get up at the same times, seven days a week. Eat at roughly the same time each day, and don't vary your diet widely from day to day so your gut can prepare effectively the enzymes it needs to digest food efficiently. Exercise at about the same time each day as well. Even meditation is best done at a consistent time daily. Respecting the "rhythm of life" can go a long way in providing emotional stability and a sense of physical well-being.

GROUP THERAPY/SUPPORT GROUPS

The presence of others can be invaluable in learning to cope with mutual problems such as phobias, anxiety, gambling, drinking, sexual addictions, anger management, and violence. These groups often prove to be one of the most affordable ways to seek professional help because they are usually led by a trained mental health worker or physician. The secret to the success of such groups seems to lie in the safety and support they provide. A person can confide long-troubling problems to others without fear of ridicule or shame. Peers can offer sympathy, caring, and support that goes far to soothing emotional upsets.

BIOFEEDBACK

Biofeedback operates on the notion that we all possess the innate ability to exert control over the automatic functions of our body through the exertion of the will and mind. A variety of instruments that monitor various body systems are used to train us to utilize and develop our mind–body connections to control anxiety and panic symptoms. The electromyogram (EMG) measures muscle tension. Two electronic sensors are placed over the muscle to be monitored. Biofeedback practitioners will most commonly use the glabellar and frontalis muscles in the fore-head, the masserter muscle of the jaw, and the trapezius muscle in the neck and upper back. In anxiety and stress management, the EMG is used to promote relaxation in muscles that have become tense in response to stress. In what is known as the body–mind connection, the relaxation of the body leads to a more relaxed and positive state of mind. The EMG works by transforming the tension signals in the muscles into a light or sound signal so you can hear or see your muscle activity. Once you are made aware of the degree of tension, your mind can learn how to allow relaxation to occur.

Temperature biofeedback uses a device that monitors skin temperature. Usually the sensor is placed on your hand or foot. During anxiety and stress, skin temperature drops as blood is redirected to the muscles and internal organs. Learning to redirect blood back to the skin will help abort the anxiety episode and allow the relaxation response to take over.

Galvanic skin response (GSR), or electrodermal response (EDR), measures electrical conduction in the skin. A very slight electrical current (unnoticeable to you) is run through your skin. The machine measures changes in the salt and water of your sweat gland ducts. The more emotionally aroused you are, the more active your sweat glands are and the greater the electrical conductivity of your skin. The GSR is effective in treating phobias, anxiety, and excessive sweating. It is also used in the lie detection test. Athletes can use this technique to prepare for competition, making sure they are not too anxious and to calm the pregame jitters.

The electroencephalogram (EEG) monitors brain wave activity. The brain emits many electrical signals of various frequencies. A few of the frequencies that have been classified are beta (awake), alpha (calm relaxation/daydreaming), theta (light sleep), and delta (deep sleep).

Learning to enhance and amplify alpha waves through biofeedback helps achieve a more relaxed state without having to take a medication. Dr. William Barton, Ph.D., a long-time practitioner of biofeedback technology in the Bay Area, has helped many resolve their phobias through a variety of simple yet effective strategies. For instance, to help a patient get over their fear of traveling through tunnels, he taught them how to use the GSR apparatus. The basic GSR device attaches to the person's fingertips, and is able to detect minute amounts of perspiration on the skin. The more tense you are, the more perspiration is measured, and the machine emits a buzzing noise. As you become calm, the perspiration, and also the buzzing noise, diminishes. Dr. Barton accompanies the patient on a number of sessions involving driving through tunnels. The patient is instructed to practice relaxation techniques that reduce the buzzing noise while traversing the tunnel. Once he figures out how to do it with the help of the machine, the patient can accomplish relaxation and abort an anxiety attack without the help of the machine. Once a reasonable level of success and confidence has been achieved, Dr. Barton allows them to "solo" (that is, drive through the tunnel alone). As discussed earlier, "emotional" learning can only occur when we realize we can do it all by ourselves, without the help of a drug, a machine, or another person by our side. Only this deep realization both consciously and subconsciously allows true healing and long-lasting recovery from phobias. For most phobias, ten to 15 sessions of biofeedback are all that is necessary to achieve significant results.

GUIDED IMAGERY/VISUALIZATION

Imagery has been considered a healing tool in virtually all of the world's cultures and is an integral part of many religions. Navajo Indians, for example, practiced an elaborate form of imagery that encourages the subject to "see" himself as healthy. Ancient Egyptians and Greeks, including Aristotle and Hippocrates, believed that images release spirits in the brain that arouse the heart and other parts of the body. They also found that strong images of a particular disease were enough to cause its symptoms.

Imagery has been found to be very beneficial for the treatment of stress. It has been shown to effectively increase brain chemicals that have a tranquilizing effect, lowering blood pressure, heart rate, and anxiety levels. Emotive imagery and visualization are especially helpful to the treatment of phobic disorders, and are used by a variety of practitioners, including biofeedback therapists, hypnotherapists, psychotherapists, and holistic practitioners. The basic technique is that the patient is guided by the therapist to imagine the anxiety-provoking phobia while at the same time learning how to relax. Biofeedback may be used to measure the degree of relaxation and progress of the patient. Visualization techniques involve teaching people how to quiet their minds, focus, and use imagery to imagine a successful result. This has been used very effectively in professional athletes. A golfer may imagine the perfect swing and practice it repeatedly while breathing calmly and learning to relax and focus before hitting the ball. The following is an example of a self-hypnosis technique that utilizes visualization and imagery:

1. Sit comfortably with your arms and legs uncrossed.

2. Take deep breaths and relax slowly from head to toe, feeling waves of relaxation washing over you. Let your eyes close gently.

3. Take yourself to a place that contains your phobia. Visualize the object of your fear in an objective way. Be an observer, disassociated from the event that is taking place.

4. Imagine yourself performing a particular task with great ease and comfort. If you have a fear of social gatherings, imagine being the life of the party, able to converse with a variety of people from varying backgrounds.

5. Complete the activity in your mind, being completely satisfied with your performance and interpersonal skills.

6. Give yourself positive affirmations that you are capable and worthy, and slowly open your eyes.

ALTERNATIVE/COMPLEMENTARY/NATURAL REMEDIES

Many healing arts and philosophies claim to have the secret for successful treatment of phobias. We do not discount the value of any of these approaches, provided the patient has been cleared of medical conditions that might impede recovery by a thorough medical evaluation. If it helps and is affordable and safe, alternative medicine is any form of practice that is outside the realm of conventional modern medicine. It covers a broad range of healing philosophies, approaches and therapies, including naturopathy, chiropractic, ayurveda, homeopathy, traditional Chinese medicine, and acupuncture. If alternative medicine is used with or in addition to conventional medicine, it is referred to as "complimentary medicine," as the two practices complement each other. For example, Dean Ornish, founder of the Preventative Medicine Research Institute in California and best-selling author, uses lifestyle changes with medications to combat heart disease; The University of Kansas uses chiropractic manipulation under general anesthesia for painful spinal conditions; many Chinese hospitals use acupuncture to reduce pain during surgery. These are all examples of complementary medicine. Holistic medicine aims at treating the "whole person," rather than individual organ systems, through integration of the mind and body. Holistic practitioners believe that our bodies are remarkably resilient machines, capable, with some occasional prodding or intervention, of healing themselves. The importance of self-care and preventing illness is emphasized in holistic medicine. Natural medicine is any therapy that relies on the body's own healing powers, and includes herbal remedies, diet, and water therapies.

HERBAL/AYURVEDIC/HOMEOPATHIC REMEDIES

Since ancient times, man has searched for natural remedies to cure his ailments. Emotional illness, such as anxiety and depression, as well as sleep disorders, fatigue, pain, irritability, and other symptoms of a dysfunctional nervous system have been the target of these remedies. Herbal remedies, ayurvedic principles, and homeopathy are still widely used in the treatment of phobias and anxiety and mood disorders.

Herbal Remedies

The following herbal remedies are so-called not because they have been proven scientifically (that is, in carefully designed blind studies) to achieve therapeutic results, but because they are widely used in some cultures, often for centuries, for the alleviation of various forms of emotional suffering. In many cases, herbs are strong chemicals that should be monitored by a medical professional. Among the most common herbal remedies for phobia-related symptoms are the following:

- *Kava Kava*—calming effects supposedly without the depressed mood sometimes associated with tranquilizers.
- *Hyperium* (St. John's Wort)—a folk remedy for anxiety, worry, depression, and sleeping problems.
- *Valerian*—used for thousands of years in India and China as a sedative and sleep inducer.
- *Chamomile*—widely used in tea form for anxiety, nervous stomach, and relaxation.
- *Ginsengs*—this group of herbal medicines, called adaptogens, reputedly strengthens the body's ability to adapt to stress and stimulates the immune system. Gingsengs come in Asian, American, and Siberian varieties, each with a somewhat different strength and application.

Ayurvedic Remedies

Ayurveda means the science of life, and espouses the natural intelligence of all living things and the universe (which is also considered a living thing). The basic ayruvedic philosophy is that health is our natural state, and that ill health is unnatural. Nature has given our bodies the intelligence to be perfectly healthy. But when stress, inadequate nutrition, or poor sleep weakens our immune systems, we then allow disease an opportunity to make us ill. The body knows how to restore balance in these situations of illness, no matter what came along to disturb this balance. Ayurveda provides insights into how to live one's life in harmony with nature and natural laws and rhythms. It provides guidelines for an intelligently regulated diet and daily routine, as well as stress management and exercises for increased fitness and alertness.

Homeopathic Remedies

Those with phobias, as well as chronic anxiety conditions, may consider trying a homeopathic remedy, especially if you are apprehensive against medical treatments, or find they gave you side effects. Be aware that homeopathy operates from quite different assumptions and methods from mainstream medical science. The following "medications" have, as a general rule, not had the benefit of thorough empirical testing. Their efficacy is largely anecdotal. Nevertheless, the treatment of phobias is not so settled a matter from the scientific perspective that other, alternative contributions can be dismissed wholesale. For homeopaths, aconite is the remedy of choice for panic attacks, as well as anxiety that is the result of a sudden fright or shock. If you are grief stricken, the homeopath may prescribe ignatia. In situations such as stage fright, "speakers nerves," and other anticipatory and performance anxiety circumstances, gelsemium is often recommended. The homeopath will usually instruct you to begin the remedy with six-times potency and take two tablets every four to six hours, depending on the severity of the condition. Once you begin to notice an improvement, you probably will be instructed to take the medication less often, and when you see significantly better, to discontinue the treatment entirely.

In homeopathy, if you use a remedy longer than necessary, it may cause the symptoms to recur. You will also be instructed to take your remedy with a clean mouth free from drink, food, tobacco, or mouthwash.

Homeopaths have found the following remedies useful in the treatment of anxiety:

1. *Aconite* (Aconitum Napellus)—indicated for panic attacks that come on suddenly and unpredictably. The symptoms of panic may include heart palpitations, shortness of breath, a sense of doom with a fear of dying, and cold sweats.

2. *Argentum Nitricum*—indicated when anxiety develops before a big event, such as a job interview, an exam, a public speech, social engagement, marriage, and so forth.

3. *Arsenicum Album*—for hypochondriacs (those who are deeply anxious about their health) and those who are extremely concerned with order and security (perhaps leaning toward obsessive-compulsive disorder).

4. *Calcarea Carbonica*—has been used for symptoms of claustrophobia and fear of heights. It is also used for those who have a problem keeping warm, are easily fatigued, have a craving for sweets, worry too much, have a nagging dread of some impending disaster, and are easily agitated by bad news.

5. *Gelsemium*—indicated for feelings of weakness, trembling, and those paralyzed by fear or complaining of mental dullness. Many phobias have been treated with this remedy, including fear of crowds, fear of falling, and fear the heart might stop beating. It is most commonly used for anticipatory anxiety, such as a public performance, impending visit to the dentist, or anxiety before a test.

6. *Ignatia Amara*—used in sensitive individuals who are anxious because of grief, loss, disappointment, criticism, loneliness, or any emotional stress. Other indications are a defensive attitude, frequent sighing, and mood swings. It has also been used for the sensation of a lump in the throat (globus hystericus).

7. *Kali Phophoricum*—for the person who is exhausted by overwork or illness. Those who are jumpy and oversensitive, feel deep anxiety and an inability to cope, or are startled by ordinary sounds may also benefit.

8. *Lycopodium*—for those who attempt to cover an inner sense of inadequacy by putting up fronts, pretending to be something they are not. They are self-conscious and easily intimated. They have a deep fear of failure, but usually do well

once they focus on a task. This remedy is thought to reduce anxiety from mental stressors and increase self-confidence.

9. *Natrum Muriaticum*—primarily used for those who hide their emotions and have a self-protective shyness that makes them seem aloof, reserved, and private. Easily hurt and offended, they often become isolated, and are known to brood, bear grudges, and dwell on unhappy feelings. Phobias that have been treated with this compound include fear of the night, fear of robbers or intruders, and claustrophobia.

10. *Phosphorus*—indicated when the patient is "openhearted, imaginative, excitable, easily startled, and full of intense and vivid fears. Strong anxiety can be triggered by thinking of almost everything." This description certainly include features of mania and hypomania.

11. *Pulsatilla*—used in patients who are anxious, insecure, and exhibit a clinginess with a need for constant support and reassurance. They fear being alone, are easily discouraged, moody, tearful, whiny, and even emotionally childish. Pulsatilla is also used for anxiety caused by hormonal changes around the time of puberty, menstrual period, or menopause.

12. *Silicea*—indicated for those individuals who are competent and serious in what they do, yet exhibit shyness, lack of confidence, and nervousness, especially when faced with a task or job that involves scrutiny by others. Anxiety caused by public appearances, interviews, and examinations is common in these perfectionists. Silicea is used to calm this anxiety, while also reducing exhaustion and increasing mental focus and concentration.

13. *Coffea Cruda*—used for jittery nerves, racing thoughts, and mental exhaustion.

TRADITIONAL CHINESE MEDICINE

Traditional Chinese medicine (TCM) is one of the oldest written medicinal systems, using herbs in conjunction with a dualistic Taoist philosophy of yin and yang. Yin (the cool, dim, yielding, and feminine component) and yang (the warm, bright, dominant, and masculine component) are viewed as the two opposing forces in all living things. In order to enjoy good health and physical and emotional harmony, every human being in the TCM perspective must maintain a balance of yin and yang. Stress and anxiety can lead to a depletion of the yin component, which can be restored with a combination of herbs, dietary adjustments, qigong exercises (incorporating deep breathing, stretching, and balancing), massage, and acupuncture. The many combinations of herbs used in TCM are designed to maintain the proper balance necessary to promote health by preventing illness.

AROMATHERAPY

Aromatherapy means "treatment using scents." It is a holistic treatment using pleasant smelling botanical oils to care for the body and improve the state of mind. Rose, lemon, lavender, and peppermint are common essential oils that may be added to a bath, massaged into the skin, inhaled directly, or diffused to scent an entire room. Aromatherapy may be used to energize, stimulate, and invigorate, or to relax, calm, and prepare for sleep. They are most commonly used to reduce anxiety and promote relaxation. When inhaled, they work on the brain and nervous system through direct stimulation of the olfactory nerve, which is evolutionarily the oldest and most primitive of the cranial nerves. The olfactory nerve has direct connections with the hypothalamus and limbic areas, including the amygdala, which are the seat of our emotional response.

The essential oils are aromatic essences extracted from plants, flowers, trees, bark, fruits, grasses, and seeds with distinctive therapeutic, psychological, and physiological properties. There are about 150 essential oils. To get the maximum benefit, the oils should be made from raw, pure, natural products. Aromatherapy is one of the fastest growing fields in alternative medicine. It is widely used in private homes, clinics, and hospitals for a variety of applications, such as pain relief for women in labor, relieving the side effects of chemotherapy in cancer patients, and improving the energy and vigor in patients who have suffered a heart attack. Aromatherapy is also slowly making its way into mainstream society. In Japan, engineers and architects are incorporating aroma systems into new buildings. In one such application, the scent of lavender and rosemary is pumped into the customer area to calm the customers waiting in line, while the perfumes from lemon and eucalyptus are used behind the counters to keep the clerks alert and responsive.

MUSIC THERAPY

Music is a significant mood-changer and reliever of stress, working on many levels at once. Many experts suggest that it is the rhythm of the music or the beat that has the calming effect on us although we may not be consciously aware of this. They point out that when we were still developing in our mother's womb, we were probably influenced by the rhythm of our mother's heartbeat. We respond to soothing music later in life, perhaps because we associate it with the safe, relaxing, and protective environment of a simpler time.

In extensive studies on what any given piece of music produces in the physiological response system, many unexpected things were found. Many of the so-called "meditation and relaxation" recordings actually produced adverse brain waves on the EEG, just as bad as hard rock and heavy metal. Surprisingly, many selections of Celtic and Native American music, as well as music containing loud drums or freely improvisational flute were extremely soothing. The most profound finding was that any music performed live, even if discordant or played at moderately loud volumes, had a very beneficial response. Whenever the proper sounds for an individual were experienced, remarkable right–left brain hemisphere synchronization occurred. The normal voltage spiking pattern coming from the brain changed to a smooth sinusoidal waveform and the usual voltage differential equalized. There were also clear benefits when the music was being created and played by the individual being studied.

Among the many stress-reducing effects of music is the increase in deep breathing that occurs when we are focused on a particular piece. Brain serotonin levels also begin to increase. Music was found to reduce the heart rate and increase core body temperature, an indication of the relaxation response. Stress is reduced by background music, even if the listener is unaware it is playing. This is why music is often piped into elevators or telephones on hold. Music also reduces anxiety and increases the pain threshold during medical procedures, and a headset is a common fixture in the modern dental office. The airlines offer a varied selection of music to keep the passengers relaxed and distracted from their fear of flying.

Here are a few recommendations for helping you create your own music therapy program. Remember, the same type of music does not work for everybody because people have different tastes. The important thing is that you choose music you like.

1. To wash away stress, try a 20-minute "sound bath." Put some enjoyable, relaxing music on the stereo, and lie near the speakers in a comfortable position on the floor or a couch. To help you focus and avoid distractions, it may be best to wear headphones.

2. Choose music with a slow rhythm—slower than your natural heartbeat. Music with a cyclical or repeating pattern is effective for most people.

3. As the music plays, imagine it flowing over you, washing away all the frustration and stress of the day. Focus on your breathing and let it slow and deepen. Focus on the silence between phrases (this keeps you from analyzing the music and makes relaxation more complete).

4. If you need to be energized and stimulated due to a sense of exhaustion and fatigue, choose a more rapid, upbeat tempo to which you can dance or tap your foot.

5. Familiarity often helps the calming response. Choose an old favorite that you know by heart.

6. Try combining exercise and imagery to your experience of music. Take a brisk walk with your favorite tunes playing on the Walkman. Inhale and exhale in rhythm with the music. Sing or hum if you like. Imagine yourself being taken to whatever fun and relaxing place the music is leading you.

7. Listen to the sounds of nature, such as the pound of the ocean surf, the calm and quiet of a deep forest, the drone of bees or other flying insects, the sound of wind rushing through the grass or rustling the tree leaves, the singing of the birds, the sound of a peaceful stream, or the falling of the rain on a canopy of jungle vegetation. If you don't have time to experience these sounds in nature, they can be found on tapes and CDs in many music stores.

PET THERAPY

The therapeutic use of pets to reduce anxiety and improve the outcome in patients with physical and emotional illnesses has gained increasing attention in recent years. For people of all ages with all kinds of problems, pets provide a constant source of comfort and focus for attention. Animals bring our nurturing instinct and make us feel safe and unconditionally accepted. We can just be ourselves, without worrying about scrutiny or unrealistic expectations or demands. Pets shift our focus away from ourselves and our problems and help us feel connected to a larger world. Surprisingly, it does not matter what type of pet—all pets have similar therapeutic value if the animal is of interest to you. The pet should be selected to fit your temperament, living space, and lifestyle.

Research has shown that exposure to pets can:

1. *Reduce stress and tension before surgery.* It was found in one study that patients who spent a few minutes watching fish before dental surgery were more relaxed as measured by their blood pressure, muscle tension, and behavior than those who did not watch the fish. In fact, patients who watched the fish were as calm as another group that had been hypnotized before surgery.

2. *Reduce blood pressure.* One study showed that the simple act of petting a dog can lower blood pressure.

3. *Boost mood and increase social interaction in the elderly.* Bringing a pet into a nursing home or hospital has been shown to effectively improve the emotional well-being of elderly and institutionalized individuals.

4. *Decrease the need for medical care.* A study conducted at UCLA found that dog owners required much less medical care for stress-related symptoms than non-dog owners.

5. *Improve the outcome after a heart attack.* A study of 92 patients hospitalized in a coronary care unit for angina or heart attack found that those who owned pets were more likely to be alive one year later than those who did not. The study found that only 6 percent of the patients who owned pets died within one year compared with 28 percent of those who did not own pets. In fact, having a pet was found to give a higher boost to the survival rate than having a spouse or a good friend!

HUMOR THERAPY

Laughing has been found to lower blood pressure, reduce the secretion of stress hormones from the adrenal glands, increase oxygen delivery to the muscles, and boost immune system elements such as the infection-fighting T-cells, disease-fighting gamma-interferon proteins, and antibody producing B-cells. Laughing also triggers endorphin release from the brain, which reduces pain and produces a general sense of well-being. Unfortunately, we often loose our sense of humor when we are anxious or depressed—just the time it is most needed. Laughter is a powerful tool to quiet the mind's overactive thought processes, thereby clearing the head of obsessive patterns of worry and fear. Rent a funny movie or stand-up comedy act. Hang out with your funniest, most upbeat friends. Think back on funny memories from your past. Start creating a scrapbook of things you find particularly hilarious. Try making others laugh by creating or learning jokes or funny stories.

HYDROTHERAPY

Hydrotherapy is the use of water in the treatment of disease. Hydrothermal therapy additionally uses the temperature effect, as in hot baths, saunas, wraps, etc. These therapies have been used in many cultures, including those of ancient Rome, China, and Japan. The ancient Greeks made therapeutic baths a way of life. Water is also an important ingredient in the traditional Chinese and Native American healing systems. A Bavarian monk, Father Sebastian Kneipp, helped repopularize the therapeutic use of water in the 19th century. There are now dozens of methods that apply hydrotherapy, including mineral baths, hot and cold showers, steam therapy, wet saunas, douches, body wraps and packs, hot and cold moist compresses, sitz baths, and footbaths.

The recuperative and healing properties of hydrotherapy are based on its mechanical and thermal effects. It exploits the body's response to hot and cold stimuli, to the protracted application of heat, to pressure exerted by the water, and to the sensation it gives. The many different specialized superficial nerves then carry impulses felt in the skin deeper into the body to the spinal reflexes and to the brain, where they are instrumental in stimulating the immune system, influencing the production of stress hormones from the adrenal glands, invigorating the circulation and digestion, encouraging blood flow, and reducing pain sensitivity.

Generally, heat quiets and soothes the body, slowing down the activity of the internal organs. Cold, in contrast, stimulates and invigorates, increasing internal activity. If you are experiencing tense muscles and anxiety, a hot shower or bath is in order. If you are feeling tired, lethargic, and stressed out, you might want to try taking a warm shower or bath, followed by a short, invigorating cold shower to help stimulate your body and mind.

Massage/Reflexology/Acupuncture (Body–Mind Approach)

A number of therapies work on the body to elicit changes in the emotions and mind. There is good neurological basis for this approach. It appears that relaxation of the body leads to relaxation of the mind, just as the relaxation response in the mind leads to decreased tension in the muscles of the body. It's just the way we are wired, and the benefits go both ways. Massage therapy, which works directly to relax the muscles by stretching them, is the second oldest form of body–mind work (sex being the oldest form). Reflexology works on the principle of pressure points in the feet, which are thought to trigger improved stimulation and therefore functioning to the body, organs, and mind. Acupuncture uses fine, disposable needles to stimulate a neurochemical response, which causes a correction in the functioning of the body while creating an increased sense of calm and well-being in the mind.

Massage therapy is the systematized manipulation of soft tissues for the purpose of normalizing them. Practitioners use a variety of physical methods, including applying fixed or movable pressure, holding, or causing stretching or movement to the body. Therapists primarily use their hands, but may also use there forearms, elbows, or feet. Touch is the core ingredient of massage, and combines science and art. Practitioners learn a variety of massage techniques and use their sense of touch to determine the right amount of pressure to be applied to each person, while also locating areas tension and other soft-tissue problems. Touch also conveys a sense of caring, an important component in the healing relationship. When muscles are overworked, or when emotional stress causes tension to build up in the muscles, waste products such as lactic acid can accumulate, causing soreness, stiffness, and even spasm. Massage improves circulation, increases blood flow, brings fresh oxygen to the tissues, and helps speed the elimination of waste products. This speeds healing after injury and can enhance recovery from disease. Therapeutic massage can be used to promote well-being and increase self-esteem while boosting the circulation and immune systems. It has been incorporated into many health systems, and different massage techniques have been developed and integrated into various complementary therapies.

HYPNOSIS/EXPOSURE THERAPY UNDER HYPNOSIS

Hypnotherapy is of particular value to those suffering from phobias. Research has shown that exposure therapy can be conducted effectively during hypnosis sessions. In effect, the therapist helps the patient achieve a deep sense of relaxation. Once the state of relaxation is achieved, the patient is guided through their feared stimulus and told to observe passively and dispassionately. The patient learns to stay calm and relaxed as they work through the phobic experience. When this has been accomplished successfully under hypnosis, the patient will find exposure therapy more tolerable.

BREATHING EXERCISES

Deep-breathing exercises are at the core of many meditative arts, and are a fundamental component of eliciting the relaxation response. When performing these exercises, one may be seated in a relaxed position, or by actively moving and stretching as with yoga. As you breathe in fully, think of the breath as your whole life that you are bringing deep into your body, including all your fears, worries, and concerns. Your slow and controlled exhalation is a metaphor for letting go of all the heavy baggage of your life, including unrealistic expectations, hurtful thoughts and emotions, and the disappointments and frustrations that poison our ability to enjoy our life in the present moment.

PRAYER/SPIRITUAL APPROACHES

Millions of human beings around the world rely regularly on prayer and other spiritual forms of meditation for the amelioration of emotional suffering, including phobias. The theological basis of such attempts at communication with the divine certainly exceeds the limits of this book. Suffice it to say that if prayer or other spiritual disciplines have proven calming and restorative to you, there is no reason why they should not play a role in your personal "anxiety toolbox." The alarms that go off when prayer is mentioned in a secular context stem from the efforts of some people to impose their own way of praying or worshipping on others.

HELPFUL MOTTOS

Security and safety is an illusion. Many spend a great deal of time and energy building a fortress around them to insulate them from the perceived threats and ugliness of the outside world. They build up reserve funds in multiple accounts in case there is a disaster, and have invested often in elaborate schemes in the aim of self-preservation. The problem is, after all is in place, they still have an overwhelming sense of fear and apprehension. That's because they have only worked on the outer, window-dressing aspects of their life and not on the tools needed to be truly fearless, confident, and comfortable in the world.

Life is not all about you. One of the quickest ways to put life problems into perspective is to take yourself out of the equation. Although the formative years of our lives are all about us—what we need and want—there comes a time when we have taken in enough from the world and it is time to give it back. Letting go of ourselves and putting the needs of others first is a basic principle of many philosophies and religious thought. In losing ourselves, we find our true self. There is no better way to strip away the layers of pretension and false values and find the calm, happy, and contented inner self that has been waiting patiently for us to be quiet and listen. Stop demanding that the world, your work, and your family exist to serve your needs. Have faith that your needs will be met if you surrender your life to the service of others.

You don't "find" happiness. The problem with happiness is that it disappears every time you start looking for it. As one wag put it, "Happiness is remembered, not experienced." In truth, happiness is both a choice and a way of life. It is not something that is delivered to your door or given to the winning lottery ticket holder. It is something that must be developed over time through consistently healthy life choices. Choosing friends and relationships wisely is of primary importance. After this, we should strive to better ourselves, not only in our work and professional careers, but also how we behave in our personal and family lives. By first making healthy, positive choices in all aspects of our lives we are preparing ourselves for a life of contentment, free from anxiety, worry, frustration, resentment, regret, and disappointment.

Let go of "status anxiety." As we achieve a certain measure of success in life, it is natural that we start thinking about how we compare and measure up to others around us. Alain de Botton, in his book *Status Anxiety* (Pantheon, 2004), notes that status anxiety is relatively modern phenomenon: "For most of history...very few among the masses had ever aspired to wealth or fulfillment; the rest knew well enough that they were condemned to exploitation and resignation." The great movements toward democracy "altered forever the basis upon which status was accorded." As Alexis de Tocqueville observed as early as 1835, "In America, I never met a citizen too poor to cast a glance of hope and envy toward the pleasures of the rich." De Botton says that status anxiety is a worry "so pernicious as to be capable of ruining extended stretches of our lives." Keeping up with, or better yet, outdoing the Joneses, is using up more of our emotional energy and generating more stress than ever before. Do we really need the biggest house, best car, or most fashionable clothes? And what is the real cost to our lives and emotional well-being. It can't be calculated merely from the sticker price.

What about the time away from our spouses and children because of the extra work hours required to maintain our elevated status? What about the loss of our hobbies and leisure activities we are passionate about? We risk losing touch with who we are and what matters most to us in a senseless attempt to make others envy and respect us by our financial achievements. The best strategy to overcome status anxiety is to learn to accept ourselves as we are, and to have faith in ourselves while retaining our humility. Practicing humility and expressing gratitude for all we have goes a long way in relieving the anxiety caused by what we don't have when compared to our friends and neighbors. After all, status is ultimately measured by the quality of our soul, not our pocketbook.

Life and joy exist in the here and now. One of the reasons we feel happy when we are around our pets is because we are renewed by the lesson they teach us about living joyfully in the present moment. Dogs are known for spontaneous celebrations over seemingly mundane and routine occurrences, such as surviving a bath, having their leash taken off, enjoying a good meal, or seeing their master come home after a short trip to the market. They get their whole body into the celebration—rolling over and kicking their legs in the air, letting their tail wag their body to the point of dangerous imbalances, and leaping in the air and running in tight circles. It is clear their joy is difficult for them to contain. Did we ever feel this way about anything? Perhaps we haven't celebrated joy since the time we were very small, before we had much of a past or were aware of a future. And that's the secret of the dog's exuberance. He is free of past regrets and has no concern about the future.

Imagine if there were no bills, no concern of where your next meal was coming from, no worry about providing for retirement, no IRS, no fear of death. Imagine if we never let past transgressions hurt us personally, scarring our self-esteem or causing disillusionment about the goodness of the universe. Of course, a dog will respond similarly to humans in burdening itself with dysfunctional anxiety and fear if it is abused or neglected. And, like us, it has a strong ability to forgive and heal when placed in a loving and stable environment. It is often said by the parents of children who are mentally challenged that these kids are special gifts in their lives. This, in part, derives from their freedom from past disappointments and future worries, allowing an unobstructed and uncluttered view of the present that is not available to most of us.

Some of you may bluntly counter that the present sucks. Why live in the present moment if you are in an unhappy marriage, just lost your job, have a family member who is ill or dying, or feel hopeless with depression. It's easier to drown the present in alcohol or blur it with drugs. Others escape to distracting activities, such as gambling, excessive exercise, home remodeling projects, or even the movies. The problem is that the real world is still there when you get back from distractions, and real problems still have to be dealt with. You only make an impact on your future by living fully and being engaged entirely in this present moment. Disappointment and loss are a part of life. We cannot grieve, heal, move on, learn new skills, and improve our lot in life unless we take full advantage of our time in the here and now.

People are more forgiving than you think. A basic misconception of many phobic sufferers is that others tend to view them harshly and scrutinize them with the hope of finding some fault or defect. In reality, most people want to stand up for the underdog and give those who have failed or fallen out of favor a second chance. On the one hand we all tend to feel better about our own defective lives when we focus on the problems of others. But, at the same time, we also want to give others a break, because we know we could easily be in the same boat some time in the future. People want to forgive and accommodate, but you must be open and trusting enough to let them.

Great courage often involves fear. Admitting fear is one of the most courageous things we can do. Most people who are recognized for courageous acts "above and beyond the call of duty" admit that they were frightened and nervous. Facing a phobia, or any emotional problem, takes tremendous courage, and anxiety and fear are signs that you have a normal, healthy emotional reaction to facing the unknown.

40 Rules to Live By in Extinguishing Anxiety

1. Get up on time every morning so you can start the day unrushed.
2. Go to bed each night at about the same time.
3. Don't accept extra projects or activities that will detract from the time you need to organize your own affairs.
4. Say *no* to friends who try to convince you to do things that help their program to the detriment of yours.
5. Pace yourself. Spread out your tasks over a reasonable timetable.
6. Delegate tasks to capable others.
7. Simplify and unclutter your life. Clean out your desks, garages, and closets, throwing out or giving away all of what you truly don't need.
8. Less is more.
9. Allow extra time to do things or get to places. Don't plan too much for one day or race to get there.
10. Take one day at a time and use it efficiently.
11. Separate worries from concerns. If you have a concern that is making you worry, ask yourself what you can do about it. If it is not something under your control, forget it. If it is something that can be resolved with your efforts, make a plan to address the problem. In any case, let go of the anxiety and worry attached to the problem and focus this wasted emotional energy on considering your options.
12. Live within your budget. Work toward a position of no debt by paying off all your credit cards and curbing all unnecessary expenses.
13. Pray, meditate, and spend time alone each day.
14. Keep your mouth shut. You don't always have to be right. Radio's Tony Grant has a trademark expression: "Would you rather be right or loved?"
15. Have backups—keep an extra car key in your wallet and an extra house key in the garden, backup important data on your computer, have extra stamps on hand, keep extra cash

for emergencies in a safe place, have a back-up list of your important addresses and phone numbers, etc.

16. Do something you enjoy every day.

17. Get regular exercise.

18. Eat right.

19. Overdo organization.

20. Write down insights and inspirations immediately. Keep a folder of quotes, scriptures, or sayings that have particular meaning to you and read them when you feel anxious.

21. Chose friends carefully. Make sure that neediness on either side is not a factor.

22. Don't waste time.

23. Laugh.

24. Take your work seriously, but not yourself.

25. Develop a forgiving attitude.

26. Be kind, even to unkind people.

27. Don't let your ego control your words or actions.

28. Apologize when you have made a mistake.

29. Express gratitude at every opportunity.

30. Talk less; listen more.

31. Slow down.

32. Remind yourself that you are not the general manager of the universe, and life is not all about you.

33. Say "thank you" and return kindnesses promptly (it's a karma thing).

34. Be humble and treat others with respect (also a karma thing).

35. Stop looking for happiness. Let it find you.

36. Give yourself a break. You don't have to be perfect. Let go of expectations that lead to frustration and unhappiness.

37. Let go of being emotionally attached to the outcome. Do your best to make thing go your way, but if the result is not what you hoped for, move on.

38. Love yourself.

39. Seek the peace through compromise.

40. Enjoy the success and talents of others.

Chapter 10

PHASING OUT YOUR PHOBIAS

This chapter answers seven questions:

1. How can you arrange for an initial evaluation and diagnosis of your condition?
2. What does it mean to "own" your phobia as an early step to recovery?
3. What primary avoidance and secondary safety behaviors are associated with your phobia?
4. How can you determine and assess forms of self-medication you have used in an attempt to relieve phobic suffering?
5. How can you evaluate the impact of phobias on your life and relationships?
6. How can you identify stressors that feed your phobias?
7. What coping skills, strategies, and tools are best suited to your needs in phasing out your phobias entirely?

So let's assume you've read this book and have concluded that you definitely have a phobia. What's more, you have resolved to take responsibility for your problem and seek a healthy, life-affirming solution. This chapter shows how to "phase out the phobia" by working on personal changes from the foundation up. Building a sound and strong base for your emotional health will not only resolve your phobia, but make you resistant to anxiety conditions for the rest of your life.

Take, for example, the story of Madeline. She came to us after many years of living with anxiety that had entered her life several times in different manifestations. What she described as "her troubles" surfaced first in high school, when she felt excessive shyness and a morbid fear of public speaking. She had actually fainted during a presentation in front of her classmates. In college, stressed by academic struggles, she developed panic attacks and had to drop out after her second year. In her early 30s, with two children and a stressful marriage, Madeline found that her inner anxiety was causing several strange behaviors, such as washing her hands excessively, constantly arranging the house so nothing was ever out of place, and making sure doors and windows were checked regularly—sometimes dozens of times a day—to make sure they were locked and secure. Over time, she had developed low self-esteem, lost her few close friends, and was barely enduring unhappy relationships with her husband and children. She was severely depressed, crying frequently, worrying incessantly, and thinking more and more about suicide. She would awaken at night with panic attacks and could not find any reason to get out of bed in the morning.

On the first visit, it became clear that Madeline had a very stressful childhood. Growing up in a strict Catholic household, she had been repeatedly molested by an older brother, who suffered from a learning disorder and depression. Her mother had turned a deaf ear to her accusations, dismissing them as evil fantasies of a young girl. The fear of having no control over her environment as well as a genetic predisposition to emotional illness would prove to be the faulty foundation leading to a lifetime of emotional dysfunction. Now that dysfunction threatened to bring down her entire life. She began the difficult process of healing by identifying the past traumas, validating her legitimate feelings of fear and anger, and learning about the cognitive distortions that had resulted from her various traumas. Madeline needed to start over, taking apart the faulty behaviors, painful personal history, and flawed beliefs.

Next, she needed to call in reputable contractors, so to speak, to build her emotional foundation with a sound design and strong materials. Family and marriage counseling, cognitive behavioral therapy, and group therapy were at the core of this new construction. Some of the underlying vulnerability would also need to be stabilized with medication, in the same way that a structure is retrofitted to make it earthquake-proof. All this would take time, resources, family cooperation, and professional insight.

If you saw Madeline today, you'd notice something that those who knew her in past years had never seen before: her engaging and confident smile.

She's literally a new person. Her dysfunctional thought patterns, chemical imbalances, and inflamed emotional brain centers have been replaced by functional thoughts, corrected imbalances, and quieted emotional responses. These are real chemical and anatomic brain changes that don't happen overnight, but can be accomplished with a team effort and Madeline's deep desire to be well.

INITIAL STEPS TOWARD PHASING OUT YOUR PHOBIA

To prepare for your individualized, integrative program to defeat your phobia, you must first gather some data and perform a few tasks:

1. **Make an appointment with your general doctor or psychiatrist and a psychologist or therapist. Like an emergency, you want to dial 911 (so to speak) first and get help on the way.**

In the meantime, while you are figuratively waiting for the paramedics to arrive, you can do your best to stabilize the situation. We recommend that you purchase the Anxiety Toolbox Program available as a download at *www.anxietytoolbox.com*. It will provide a step-by-step framework that is easy to follow, even if you are very busy. In addition, you can complete the Comprehensive Anxiety Screening Tool (CAST) self-test included in the program. Just print out the result to take with you to your first visit with the doctor and therapist. Filling out the following section will prepare you well for the Anxiety Toolbox Program and set you on the path to freedom from disruptive phobias or any other anxiety conditions.

Choosing a physician that is knowledgeable about phobias may be a challenge. Even if your doctor is not comfortable treating anxiety or phobia conditions, a basic medical evaluation should be done first anyway. If this examination proves normal, the physician may then refer you to a qualified psychiatrist, if needed. Choosing a psychologist or therapist can be equally daunting. You can ask your physician for a referral or have your insurance company provide a list of qualified therapists on your plan. If you don't like the first one you meet, try another. Talk with friends who have had successful therapy experiences and ask for an introduction to their doctor.

Doctor appointment   date: _____ time: _____

Therapist appointment date: _____ time: _____

2. **The next step is to accept and "own" your phobias and other emotional disorders.**

Put aside for now the blame that can be placed on others for your problems. Acknowledge that it is your responsibility to work toward gaining understanding and control of these problems. Also recognize that by doing so you are not only improving the quality of your life, but the lives of all those who depend on you or come in contact with you. Accomplishing physical and emotional health is our obligation as responsible human beings, and it is the first rule of many great religions and paths of spiritual growth (for example, treating your mind and body as a temple). Without this health we are a burden to others rather than a blessing. Make a decision now that your first priority in life is to work on building a strong foundation of physical and emotional health, and that every lifestyle decision will be informed by this ultimate goal and priority. List the problems that you agree to own, including your phobia and any other disorder diagnosed by a physician or suspected by you based on what you have read:

My phobia is: _____

My anxiety disorder(s) is/are: _____

My mood disorder is: _____

My personality disorder is: _____

My substance abuse/overuse condition(s) is/are: _____

_____

I fear the following external activities, situations, and places: _____

_____

The first sign of an impending symptom attack are the following feelings or sensations: _____

_____

My symptom attack can best be described as: _____

_____

My feared catastrophe is: _____

_____

3. **Identify your primary avoidance and secondary safety behaviors:**

Some of my avoidance behaviors are: _____

_____

Some of my safety behaviors are:

_____

_____

4.   **List any forms of "self-medication."**

In this case, we are referring to negative or potentially harmful substances or activities that you have turned to now or in the past to reduce
anxiety, help you sleep, or avoid facing your problems or fears. Self-
medication could include drugs such as alcohol, nicotine, or marijuana,
or the excessive pursuit of an activity that distracts us from our fears,
like overexercising, overeating, gambling, or overindulging in sexual
interests. The forms of self-medication we are talking about lead us further from insight and control and may compound our stress by intro-
ducing new health, legal, financial, or social problems into our lives:

In an attempt to feel better, I have used the following means of
self-medication: _____

_____

5.   **List the ways this phobia and the accompanying avoidance and
      safety behaviors have impacted your life:**

My phobia has affected the relationship with my spouse/significant
other in the following ways:

_____

_____

My phobia has affected other relationships (kids, boss, coworkers,
and friends) in the following ways:

_____

_____

My phobia has affected my career in the following ways:

_____

6.   **What factors, in your mind, contributed to the development of
      this phobia in your case?**

Think of your genetics, temperament, negative parenting, childhood
peer influences, embarrassing conditioning experiences, or traumatic
experiences occurring in adulthood:

_____

_____

7.   List your greatest stressors.

Include unhealthy lifestyle choices, destructive relationships, work and family stress, financial worries, and health problems. Write down next to each stressor the ways in which you can exert control over this problem. Many people feel they are in a rut with family-, financial-, or work-related issues. Discuss these difficulties with your family and counselor and look for areas of self-induced stress. Are you creating stress through a bad habit, unrealistic expectation, from failing to control a situation that requires your assertiveness, or from attempting to control a situation that you should not or cannot control? The more you gain insight into your stress, the more you will be able to disentangle yourself from it:

8.   What anxious cognitions intensify, magnify, or maintain your phobia?

After reading this book, do you recognize any misperceptions or misinterpretations that feed into your phobia?

Now that you have identified your problems, you have the ability to create a program to overcome them. But first, let's think about our game plan by calling to mind the assets, skills, and tools you already possess or can acquire to wage a successful battle.

9.   What positive attributes, tools, or coping skills do have to control this phobia, and what are your strengths, belief system, and support system?

Think about things you already know, have, or do. For example, perhaps you already eat right, exercise, and meditate. Perhaps you have a positive relationship with a spouse or friend, or other forms of family and social support. Perhaps you have a good job with little or no financial worries. Perhaps you are a kind, thoughtful, good-hearted, intelligent, insightful, experienced, or talented individual. You may bring a strong set of values or spiritual beliefs to help combat your fears.

10. What lifestyle changes would be helpful in reducing anxiety?

Think about the changes that would allow better sleep, diet, and exercise. What changes would reduce your overall stress by simplifying and organizing your living space and financial life? How could you stop destructive behaviors and replace them with health-affirming activities? Are there any relationships that do not support your new, healthy direction (such as friends that insist on using drugs, gambling, etc., and are always trying to get us to partake in or support these habits)? What professional help, such as your doctor, attorney, or financial planner, will be necessary? If you can't afford this help, do you have any family or community resources that can be called upon for advice?

---

11. What tools appeal to you in building an integrative strategy to phase out the phobia?

Look through Chapter 9 and list those tools you would be willing to learn or try:

---

12. What strategies have your doctor, psychiatrist, psychologist, or counselor recommended?

Include medications, stress management, cognitive behavioral therapy, or any other modalities:

---

13. Finally, write down your personal reasons for wanting to overcome your phobia and other conditions that are affecting your life:

Using the previous insights, observations, and professional advice, you are now ready to embark on the path to freedom from fear. This path will require that we continually challenge your deeply held misconceptions and expose you to your fears in a scientific and controlled way. The cornerstone of successful treatment of phobias is exposure to what is feared. *In vivo* exposure means confronting something in real life. This is the most successful form of treatment for phobias, and requires that you gradually expose yourself to real-life situations that involve the object of your phobic fear. Another form of exposure therapy, called *interoceptive exposure*, involves exposing yourself to internal sensations and feelings that trigger your anxiety.

As stated at the outset of this book, overcoming your phobia will require the involvement of both the rational and emotional elements of your mind. The Anxiety Toolbox Program will guide you through these cognitive corrections and exposure experiences in a supportive and organized fashion. It will further encourage positive lifestyle choices, stress management, and the affirmation of sound, healthy decision-making skills. Along the way, you will also be adding tools to your toolbox—the tools you will need to build a new foundation for your emotional health.

We want to congratulate you for coming this far on the journey to end your phobia. We are confident that with your continued courage and support as needed from health professionals, you will cross the finish line as a regenerated, happy, and phobia-free person.

Note: For an organized, interactive, and inspiring day-by-day approach to overcoming phobias or any other anxiety condition, you can purchase as a download the Anxiety Toolbox Program at *www.anxietytoolbox.com*. You will also find the most comprehensive self-test available anywhere for identifying anxiety disorders, created exclusively for this online program. It will help you and your doctor arrive at the most accurate diagnosis.

REFERENCES AND RECOMMENDED READING

Ainsworth. "Attachment: Retrospect and Prospect." In *The Place of Attachment in Human Behavior*, by Parks and Stevenson-Hinde, 3–30. New York: Basic Books, Inc., 1982.

American Psychiatric Association. *Diagnostic and Statistical Manual of Mental Disorders, DSM-IV*. Washington, D.C.: American Psychiatric Association, 2000.

Amering, M., et al. "Embarrassment About the First Panic Attack Predicts Agoraphobia in Panic Disorder Patients." *Behavior Research and Therapy* 35(6) (1997): 517–521.

Barlow, D. *Mastery of Your Anxiety and Panic II*. San Antonio, Tex.: Graywind Publications, 1994.

Barrett, P.M., R.M. Rapee, and M.R. Dadds. "Family Treatment of Childhood Anxiety: A Controlled Trial." *J. Consult. Clin. Psychol.* 64 (1996): 333–342.

Bassett, L. *From Panic to Power*. New York: HarperResource, 1997.

Blehar, M.C., A.F. Lieberman, and M.D.S. Ainsworth. "Early Face-to-Face Interaction and Its Relation to Later Infant–Mother Attachment." *Child Dev.* 48 (1977): 182–194.

Bourne, E. *The Anxiety & Phobia Workbook, 3rd edition*. Oakland, Calif.: New Harbinger Publications, 2000.

———*Beyond Anxiety & Phobia*. Oakland, Calif.: New Harbinger Publications, 2001.

Brown, D. *Flying Without Fear*. Oakland, Calif.: New Harbinger Publications, 1996.

Bruch, M. "Familial and Developmental Antecedents of Social Phobia: Issues and Findings." *Clin. Psychol. Rev.* 9 (1989): 37–47.

Butler, G. *Overcoming Social Anxiety and Shyness*. New York: New York University Press, 2001.

Calkins, S.D., N.A. Fox, and T.R. Marshall. "Behavioral and Psychological Antecedents of Inhibited and Uninhibited Behavior." *Child Dev.* 67 (1996): 523–540.

Caster, Inderbitzen, and Hope. "Relationship Between Youth and Parent Perceptions of Family Environment and Social Anxiety." *J. Anxiety Disord.* 13 (1999): 237–251.

Cooper, P.J., and M. Elke. "Childhood Shyness and Maternal Social Phobia: A Community Study." *Br. J. Psychiatry* 174 (1999): 439–443.

Craske, M. et al. "Interceptive Exposure Versus Breathing Retraining in Cognitive-Behavioral Therapy for Panic Disorder With Agoraphobia." *British Journal of Clinical Psychology* 36 (1997): 85–99.

Davidson R. "Asymmetric Brain Function, Affective Style, and Psychopathology: The Role of Early Experience and Plasticity." *Dev. Psychol.* 6 (1994): 741–758.

Davis, M. et al. *The Relaxation & Stress Reduction Workbook, 5th edition*. Oakland, Calif.: New Harbinger Publications, 2000.

De Botton, Alain. *Status Anxiety*. New York: Pantheon, 2004.

DeWit, D.J., A. Ogborne, D.R. Offord, and K. MacDonald. "Antecedents of the Risk of Recovery From DSM-III-R Social Phobia." *Psychol. Med.* 29 (1999): 569–582.

Dechant Jm. *Christian Yoga*. New York: HarperCollins, 2000.

Drummond, L. "Behavioral Approaches to Anxiety Disorders." *Postgraduate Medical Journal* 69(8) (1993): 222–226.

Epstein, Seymour, and Archie Brodsky. *You're Smarter Than You Think*. New York: Simon & Schuster, 1993.

Essau, C.A., J. Conradt, and F. Petermann. "Frequency and Comorbidity of Social Phobia and Social Fears in Adolescents." *Behav. Res. Ther.* 37 (1999): 831–843.

Evans. "Communicative Competence as a Dimention of Shyness." In *Social Withdrawal, Inhibition, and Shyness in Childhood*, edited by Rubin, and Asendorpf, 189–212. Hillsdale, N.J.: Lawrence Erlbaum and Associates, 1993.

Fava, G. et al. "Overcoming Resistence to Exposure in Panic Disorder With Agoraphobia." *Acta Psychiatrica Scandinavica* 95 (1997): 306–312.

Feske, and Chambless. "Cognitive-Behavioral Versus Exposure-Only Treatment for Social Phobia: A Meta-Analysis." *Behavior Therapy* 26 (1995): 695–720.

Ginsburg, La Greca, and Silverman. "Social Anxiety in Children With Anxiety Disorders: Relation With Social and Emotional Functioning." *J. Abnorm. Child Psychol.* 26 (1998): 175–185.

Gould, Buckminster, Pollack, Otto, and Yap. "Cognitive-Behavioral and Pharmacologic Treatment for Social Phobia: A Meta-Analysis." *Clinical Psychology: Science and Practice* 4 (1997): 291–306.

Graham, and Juvonen. "Self-Blame and Peer Victimization in Middle School: An Attributional Analysis." *Dev. Psychol.* 34 (1998): 587–599.

Heimberg, R.G. "Cognitive-Behavioral Therapy for Social Anxiety Disorder." *Biological Psychiatry* 51 (2002): 101–108.

Heimberg, Dodge, Hope, Kennedy, Zollo, and Becker. "Cognitive Behavioral Group Treatment for Social Phobia: Comparison With Acredible Placebo Control." *Cognitive Therapy and Research.* 14 (1990): 1–23.

Heimberg, and Juster. "Cognitive-Behavioral Treatments: Literature Review." In *Social Phobia, Diagnosis, Assessment, and Treatment*, edited by Heimberg, Liebowitz, Hope, and Schneier, 261–309. New York: Guilford Press, 1995.

Kendler, K.S., M. Neale, R. Kessler, A. Heath, and L. Eaves. "The Genetic Epidemiology of Phobias in Women: The Interrelationship of Agoraphobia, Social Phobia, Situational Phobia, and Simple Phobia." *Arch. Gen. Psychiatry* 49 (1992): 273–281.

Kendler, K.S., E. Walters, M. Neale, R. Kessler, A. Heath, and L. Eaves. "The Structure of the Genetic and Environmental Risk Factors for Six Major Psychiatric Disorders in Women." *Arch. Gen. Psychiatry* 52 (1995): 374–383.

Kendler, K.S., L.M. Karkowski, and C.A. Prescott. "Fears and Phobias: Reliability and Heritability." *Psychol. Med.* 29 (1999): 539–553.

Levinson, H. *Phobia Free*. New York: M. Evans and Company, 1988.

Lieb, R., H.U. Wittchen, M. Hofler, M. Feutsch, M.B. Stein, and K.R. Merikangas. "Parental Psychopathology, Parenting Styles, and the Risk of Social Phobia in Offspring: A Prospective Longitudinal Community Study." *Arch. Gen. Psychiatry* 57 (2000): 859–866.

Marks, I., and R. Dar. "Fear Reduction by Psychotherapies: A Response." *British Journal of Psychiatry* 177 (2000): 280.

Markway, B. et al. *Painfully Shy: How to Overcome Social Anxiety and Reclaim Your Life*. New York: St. Martin's Griffin, 2003.

McManus, F. et al., Specificity of cognitive biases in social phobia and their role in recovery. *Behavioral and Cognitive Psychotherapy* 28:201–209 (2000).

Öhmann, A., and S. Mineka. "Fears, Phobias, and Preparedness: Toward an Evolved Module of Fear and Fear Learning." *Psycholoical Review* 108(3) (2001):483–522.

Ost. "Ways of Acquiring Phobias and Outcome of Behavioral Treatments." *Behav. Res. Ther.* 23 (1985): 683–689.

Otto, M.W. "Learning and 'Unlearning' Fears: Preparedness, Neural Pathways, and Patterns." *Biological Psychiatry* 52 (2002): 917–920.

————"Cognitive-Behavioral Therapy for Social Anxiety Disorder: Model, Methods, and Outcome." *Journal of Clinical Psychiatry* 60(suppl 9) (1999): 14–19.

Peurifoy, R. *Anxiety, Phobias, & Panic: A Step-by-Step Program for Regaining Control of Your Life*. New York: Warner Books, 1995.

Pollard, C., N. Simon, and M. Otto. *Social Anxiety Disorder: Research and Practice*. New York: Professional Publishing Group, Ltd., 2003.

Pollard, C., and E. Zuercher-White. *The Agoraphobia Workbook*. Oakland, Calif.: Harbinger Publications, 2003.

Rapee, R. *Overcoming Shyness and Social Phobia*. New York: Rowman Aronson, Inc., 1998.

Rapee, R., and Heimberg. "A Cognitive-Behavioral Model of Anxiety in Social Phobia." *Behav. Res. Ther.* 35 (1997): 741–756.

Rosenbaum, J.F., J. Biederman, D.R. Hirshfeld, S.V. Faraone, E.A. Bolduc, J. Kagan, N. Snidman, and J.S. Reznick. "Further Evidence of an Association Between Behavioral Inhibition and Anxiety Disorders: Results From a Family Study of Children From a Non-Clinical Sample." *J. Psychiat. Res.* 25 (1991): 49–65.

Roth, D.A., and R.G. Heimberg. "Cognitive-Behavioral Models of Social Anxiety Disorder." *Psychiatric Clinics of North America* 24 (2001):753–771.

Schmidt, L.A., N.A. Fox, J. Schulkin, and P.W. Gold. "Behavioral and Psychophysiological Correlates of Self-Presentation in Temperamentally Shy Children." *Dev. Psychobiol.* 35 (1999): 119–135.

Schneier, F.R., J. Johnson, C.D. Hornig, M.R. Liebowitz, and M.M. Weisman. "Social Phobia: Comorbidity and Morbidity in an Epidemiological Sample." *Arch. Gen. Psychiatry* 49 (1992): 282–288.

Stahl, S. *Essential Psychopharmacology, 2nd edition*. Cambridge: Cambridge University Press, 2000.

Stein, M.B., M. Chartier, A. Hazen, M. Kozak, M. Tancer, S. Lander, P. Furer, D. Chubaty, and J. Walker. "A Direct Interview Family Study of Generalized Social Phobia." *Am. J. Psychiatry* 155 (1998): 90–97.

Stemberg, Turner, Beidel, and Calhoun. "Social Phobia: An Analysis of Possible Developmental Factors." *J. Abnormal Psychol.* 104 (1995): 526–531.

Stopa, I. "Social Phobia and Interpretation of Social Events." *Behavior Research and Therapy* 38 (2000): 273–283.

Taylor, S. "Meta-Analysis of Cognitive-Behavioral Treatments for Social Phobia." *Journal of Behavior Therapy and Experimental Psychiatry* 27 (1996): 1–9.

Weinstock, L.S. "Gender Differences in the Presentation and Management of Social Anxiety Disorder." *J. Clin. Psychiatry* 60 (suppl 9) (1999): 9–13

Wells, Clark, Salkovskis, Ludgate, Hackmann, and Gelder. "Social Phobia: The Role of In-Situation Safety Behaviors in Maintaining Anxiety and Negative Beliefs." *Behavior Therapy* 26 (1995): 153–161.

Young, E. Know *Fear: Facing Life's Six Most Common Phobias*. New York: Broadman & Holman Publishers, 2003.

INDEX

About the Authors

James Gardner, M.D., is the coauthor of *Overcoming Anxiety, Panic, and Depression* (New Page Books) and heads a large medical practice in Marin County, California. He holds degrees from Stanford University and the University of California at Los Angeles, and is a clinical instructor at the University of California at San Francisco.

Arthur H. Bell, Ph.D., is professor of management communication and director of communication programs at the Masagung Graduate School of Management, University of San Francisco. He holds his Ph.D. from Harvard University and is the author of more than 30 books focusing on management skills. He is coauthor with Dr. Gardner of *Overcoming Anxiety, Panic, and Depression* (New Page Books).